THE WHEEL OF HEALTH

THE SOURCES OF LONG LIFE AND HEALTH AMONG THE HUNZA

G. T. WRENCH

DOVER PUBLICATIONS, INC.
MINEOLA, NEW YORK

Bibliographical Note

This Dover edition, first published in 2006, is an unabridged republication of the work originally published in 1938 by the C. W. Daniel Company, Ltd., London.

International Standard Book Number: 0-486-45154-2

Manufactured in the United States of America
Dover Publications, Inc., 31 East 2nd Street, Mineola, N.Y. 11501

CONTENTS

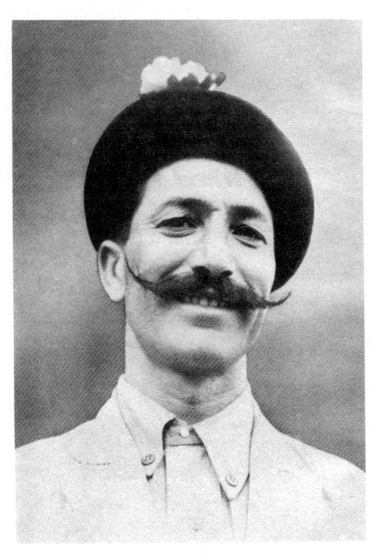

A MAN OF HUNZA

INTRODUCTION

It should be clearly understood that a doctor is one so saturated with people's illnesses and ailments that, if thoughtful, he is almost forced to look upon life as something heavily burdened by these defects.

I shall myself carry with me the profound impression of the first months I spent in the hospital wards and out-patient departments many years ago. I had come from the vigorous and exuberant life of an English public school, where everything that really absorbed one's boyish interests was based on a glowing vitality and responsive health. After the penance of school hours there was plenty of time to let the muscles go—games, sports, ragging, bathing, or running and walking over untilled fields. All these things were of sunlight and wind or the raw cold, which made the blood snap round its course.

Something of this life accompanies the early years of the medical student, but there is always about one the lure of the hospital work to draw one to its consuming interests. One is caught in the meshes of the problems of disease, from which one will not be able to free the mind for the rest of one's life.

For impressions of youth are those that remain. They colour all one's thought and experience, they largely select that thought and experience. And the impression of the quantity of diseases and the suffering due to them is a tremendous one. I used sometimes to walk about London with my eyes down and with the question "Why?" upon my lips until I saw pictures of the many maleficent objects of pathology upon the pavements, so vivid was the impression which the microscope and the post-mortem room made upon me.

The effect was not one of depression; that is not the effect upon healthy youth. It was one which stimulated one like a stouter opponent than oneself at boxing. Here was truly a prodigious opponent, the problem of disease, why man is so affected.

After debating the question—Why disease? Why not health?—again and again with my fellow students, I slowly, before I qualified, came to a further question—Why was it that as students we were always presented with sick or convalescent people for our teaching and never with the ultra-healthy? Why were we only taught disease? Why was it presumed that we knew all about health in its fulness? The teaching was wholly one-sided. Moreover, the basis of our teaching upon disease was pathology, namely, the appearance of that which is dead from disease.

We started from our knowledge of the dead, from which we interpreted the manifestations, slight or severe, of threatened death, which is disease. Through these various manifestations, which fattened our text-books, we approached health. By the time, however, we reached real health, like that of the keen times of public school, the studies were dropped. Their human representatives, the patients, were now well, and neither we nor our educators were any longer concerned with them. We made no studies of the healthy—only the sick.

Disease was the reason for our specialised existences. There was also a great abundance of it. Between its abundance and its need to ourselves its inevitability was taken for granted. Gradually, however, a question forced itself upon me more and more insistently. Had not some of this "inevitability" attached to disease come about by our profession only viewing disease from within? What would happen if we reversed the process and started by learning all we could about the healthiest people and animals whom we could discover? This question pursued me with considerable constancy, but unfortunately I was not provided with that will which is a part of what I reverence so much—the genius of discovery. Those who possess it grip an idea and never let it go. They are as passionate for it to get on in the world as the mother is for her offspring; daring, as even weak animals do, to challenge hopeless odds on its behalf. After achieving a small local repute in research, all I did was to apply for scholarships, and in my applications I placed a subject of my own choice, to study the health of the healthiest people I could discover.

I did not, of course, succeed. My proposal was probably looked upon as ridiculous. To research in health was a complete reversal of the accustomed outlook, which was confined by the nature of the profession to different aspects of disease. For to the profession disease is the base and substance of its structure and health just the top of the pyramid, where it itself comes to an end. To propose reversing this was like asking one to stand on one's head to get the right point of view.

At any rate my applications came to nothing, though I was offered work upon the accepted lines. In this I had not the necessary faith, so I gave up research and went into practice. I remained interested in very healthy people and read what I could about them, but the work imposed by the war and by practice in the following years withheld me from anything more than an academic interest in the old question—Health; why not?

It was not until two years ago, when I had more leisure, that a vivid sentence in the writings of Sir Robert McCarrison thawed my frozen hope. The sentence was: "These people are unsurpassed by any Indian race in perfection of physique; they are long lived, vigorous in youth and age, capable of great endurance and enjoy a remarkable freedom from disease in general." Further study of his writings was very encouraging. Here was a research worker who researched in health and healthy people; in fact he presented to himself health as a problem, and produced answers to it, in some such words as the following: "Here is a people of unsurpassed health and physique, and here are researches into the reasons thereof."

In this way it will be seen we come as researchers straight to health without intervention, and to health in the full dictionary sense of the word of wholeness, namely, sound physique of every organ of the body without exceptions and freedom from disease. This is the knowledge which we all want to know. We want to know what is full health, whether the tremendous part illness and ailments play in modern civilized countries is really necessary and, if not, upon what primarily does health depend. We can ourselves attain to health—or at least with our modern skill in investigation we should be able to do so—

if this full health exists in any part of our Empire to-day. We shall at least learn more about how to be healthy ourselves and how to bring healthy children into the world by studying successful human examples than we can by any other way.

By studying the wings of birds in flight we have made our machines carry us through the air. By studying one of the healthiest peoples of the world we might so improve our methods of health as to become a really healthy people ourselves. A research in health is really promising. Well, here is one. Let us see if the promise is fulfilled.

Chapter I

THE HUNZA PEOPLE

WHERE India meets Afghanistan and the Chinese Empire and is closest to the Soviet Republics, there, amidst a congress of great mountains, is the Native State of Hunza.

If one looks at a map of this part of the world with the mountain ranges shown by strongly-marked lines, they are seen to sweep towards each other to meet to the north of, at and to the south of the cleft of the Hunza valley.

A map in Mrs. Visser-Hoofts' *Among the Kara-Korum Glaciers* (1926) is of this kind. To the north is the mighty wall of the Tien-shan, coming from Mongolia, as the northern border of the Chinese Turkestan, to merge itself with the Pamir in the west, to the north of Hunza. South of the Tien-shan, forming the southern boundary of Turkestan and separating it from Tibet, is the curved line of the Kwen-lun, passing from east to west also to meet the line of the Pamir.

Yet further south, passing from west to east, is the straight line of the Hindu-Kush. From the east, passing west and meeting the Hindu-Kush at the cleft of Hunza, is the Kara-Korum range. Sweeping up from the south-east is the main Himalaya, ending in the lesser ranges of Chitral and Afghanistan to the south of Hunza.

In the congress of these huge ranges is to be found the greatest folding of the earth's surface, and where the folding is actually greatest, that is between the Hindu-Kush to the west and the Kara-Korum to the east, there, in a profound cleft, between walls of ten to fifteen thousand feet in height, lies the habitable part of Hunza.

Could any place be less like England, or London, which now harbours a quarter of England's population? Is any place less likely to give us guidance in matters of health than this cleft between its prodigious unscaled mountain walls?

9

That seems a reasonable enough doubt. Certainly there are
stupendous superficial differences. Yet, the beautiful and
highly cultivated sunny seven miles, which is the heart of
Hunza, may, by its very remoteness, have sheltered primary
truths of health which our civilisation has forgotten.

Fortunately many people have seen the Hunza folk, for their
valley is the highway to the 15,600 feet wall which divides
India from China and is called the Mintaka Pass. The pass
is itself only some ten miles from the extreme eastern corner
of Afghanistan. Moreover, a good walker, starting early in the
day, can pass over it and reach Kizil Robat, which is the most
south-eastern post of Bolshevist Asia. So a lot of people have
passed along this cleft, and no doubt in the past a lot more,
in big invading troops, would like to have done so. Actually,
more than a thousand years ago an army of ten thousand
Chinese did cross the Darkot Pass (15,400 feet) into the neighbouring valley of Yasin and occupied the Gilgit district,
but that proved to be an inimitable feat. With this exception,
these clefts have only been traversed by small groups of men.
In modern times most of the European explorers, missionaries,
and officials, on their way from India to Central Asia, take the
Hunza route.

Europeans do not live in Hunza. In transit they spend a few
days in Baltit, the capital of Hunza, collecting coolies for their
further journey and enjoying the hospitality of its famous ruler,
Mir Mohammed Nazim Khan. So there is no account of
Hunza by a resident. Nevertheless, many travellers have left
their impressions of Hunza, and the officials of the Gilgit
Agency to which Hunza is now attached, have to visit the
valley on their official rounds. Hence a good deal is known
about the Hunza people, but superficially rather than
intimately. They are still a people peculiarly themselves. They
have preserved their remoteness from the ways and habits of
the modern world, and with it those methods of life which
contribute or cause the excellent physique and bodily health
which is theirs.

The travellers and officials with one voice bear testimony
to the Hunzas' physique. They find these people not only

fearless, good-tempered and cheerful, but also as possessing a marvellous agility and endurance.

For example, that illustrious traveller and savant Sir Aurel Stein, when on the way to the "Sand-buried Ruins of Khotan" (1903), was amazed on the morning of June 25th to see a returning messenger who had been sent by the Mir to the political Munshi of Tashkurghan to prepare him for Stein's impending arrival. The messenger had started on the 18th. It was just seven complete days between his start and his return, and in that time he had travelled two hundred and eighty miles on foot, speeding along a track mostly two to four feet wide, sometimes only supported on stakes let into the cliff wall, and twice crossing the Mintaka Pass, which is the height of Mont Blanc. The messenger was quite fresh and undisturbed, and did not consider that what he had done was unusual.

Nor was it, not even its speed. To pass along mountain tracks, of course, is the only way the people can get out of their strip of green country between river and mountain. But that does not make their going up and down and across the faces of precipices easy-going. Yet "it is quite a usual thing for a Hunza man to walk the sixty miles to Gilgit at one stretch, do his business and return direct," says Colonel R. C. F. Schomberg, who for eight years had occasion to visit the Gilgit Agency and saw much of the Hunza.

They are a peculiar people, almost like the mountain ibex which they hunt, in the ease of their gait. When they traverse these huge distances they have such a quick, light way of passing over the ground that they can be detected at great distances from other peoples on a mountain track. "How can you tell at such a distance that those laden coolies are Hunza?" asked Schomberg of his native companions. "By the way they walk," was the reply.

Indeed, interpolated in the fascinating narrative of Schomberg's travels *Between the Oxus and the Indus* (1905) one finds a constant pæan of the physique and excellence of the Hunza. This is the more interesting, for Schomberg visited a number of other populated valleys of the Gilgit Agency, and, though mountainous conditions and climate were the same, the people did not compare, on the whole, in physique and quality with the Hunza.

Some of the peoples, however, Schomberg found, approached but did not reach the Hunza. He set out from Gilgit and passed through the fief of Punyal. "The Punyalis," he writes, "are splendid climbers," and then comes a little bit of the pæan, "second only to the men of Hunza."

Punyal is the first bit of country to the west, going from Gilgit, up the valley of the Gilgit river, with the mountains of Hunza on the right. Some sixty miles further westwards is Ghizr, on the borders of Chitral. The people of Ghizr are lazy. They do not store food carefully for the winter, and at the end of the winter are usually starving. Schomberg's two Hunza attendants mocked at the hovels in which the men of Ghizr lived. The owners of the hovels replied meekly that they knew their houses were squalid and miserable, but they could not be troubled to build new ones. The general assent with which the bystanders received this explanation showed how ingrained this laziness of character was in the Ghizr people. Now, the Hunza are a most industrious people. And yet Hunza and Ghizri are not far apart, and both live within similar surroundings.

Two valleys, like the Hunza in being made by rivers flowing from the Kara-Korum glaciers south to the Gilgit river, lie to the west of Hunza. The first is Ishkoman, the second Yasin. Schomberg visited both. The Yasinis had fine lands and ample crops, and were, moreover, of fine physique, though falling short of the folk of Hunza and Punyal. Yet the Ishkomanis, whose valley is between that of the Yasinis and that of the Hunza, though living under apparently like conditions to their neighbours, were poor, undersized, under-nourished creatures. There was plenty of land and water, but the Ishkomanis were too indolent to cultivate it with thoroughness, and the possibility of bad harvests was not enough to overcome their sloth. They had a number of yaks, but they were too lazy to load them or to ride them or to collect their valuable hair or even to milk them. They had no masons or carpenters or craftsmen in their country.

Many of them showed signs of disease. "The more I saw of the Ishkomanis, the more I was struck by their degeneracy; they were poor in physique and lacking in brains; a strange type of mountaineer!" (Schomberg). Why they were so poor a type with such fine people on the other side of the eastern wall of their valley their visitor does not say. But it is so. These poor Ishkomanis, who danced to entertain their guests, looked like "newly-hatched chickens," as a Hunza spectator scornfully remarked, whereas the Hunza dance is altogether wonderful, according to travellers.

The difference of the Ishkomanis and the Hunza cannot be due to their being on different sides of their twenty-thousand feet wall. In this relation the two peoples are not north and south, but west and east. Both valleys run to the south from the main range, so the similarity of their situation remains.

From the valley where "the people represent as low a type of humanity as any in north-west India" Schomberg passed from the south into the valley of the Hunza river. On the way he had to pass through the territory of one more people, the Nagiris of the Native State of Nagir, situated on the southern side of the Hunza river valley, but with a capital a little removed in a branch valley joining the main valley from the east.

The Nagiris, though facing the people of Hunza, are not of their physical class. By all travellers who write of them this is noted. They are of good physique in the main, but they fail to reach the supreme excellence and energy of the Hunza, which makes so light of the stern conditions in which both live.

It is recorded that in all the little wars that arose between these neighbours, the Hunza, though less numerous, have invariably won. Even in games it is the same. Bruce, in 1894, organised various sports and games between Hunza and Nagiris. The Hunza men won every event. As coolies for mountaineering expeditions the Hunza have greatly the superior reputation. They are superb mountaineers and unequalled slab climbers, whereas the Nagiris have no such superlative repute. Nor have the Nagiris the brightness and good humour of the Hunza; they are more sedate and morose.

The Nagiris give as a reason for this difference that in winter, when the sun is in the south, they on the south side of the valley are in the shadow of the great mountains, whereas the Hunza on the northern side enjoy the sun. It is true that, owing to a western bend to the river, the Hunza do get more sun, but this extra sun would not cover the Hunza superiority to the men of Ghizr and many others who also live on the northern side of their west to east valleys. Still, this is a difference which we, in a British winter, can appreciate.

The Nagiris are slovenly and have unclean habits, because of which, say the Hunza, they also have such swarms of flies. They are content with squalid houses and with indolent workmanship. "The people of Nagir," writes Schomberg, "are poor husbandmen, believing rather in the kindness of Providence than in hard work, and their lovely fertile country owes but little to its owners."

Passing Nagir, Hunza is reached. It is in the main a stretch of intense cultivation, extending some seven to eight miles along the northern bank of the Hunza river. It is a place of brilliant beauty. Facing it to the south is the great white cloud of Rakaposhi, 25,550 feet high, rising some 18,000 feet above the valley itself and dominating it, though on a vaster scale, as Mont Blanc dominates the valley of Chamonix. Between the valley and the snows are huge barren precipices, except where the slopes allow of terraced vegetation. These terraces in summer are bands of brilliant green or golden corn from the river bank almost up to the verge of the snows. In the autumn the green of the abundant fruit trees change to scarlet and gold and vermilion and even bright pink, so that Mr. Skrine in *Chinese Central Asia* (1926), on his way through Hunza, wonders that no artist has made his name "world-famous" by transferring to his canvas something of the incomparable brilliancy of the multi-coloured valley, with its tremendous frame of grim, rocky walls, above which are the immeasurable snows.

Here dwell the Hunza, whose numbers Major Biddulph in *Tribes of the Hindoo Koosh* (1880) roughly calculated as

6,000 people, but who have, since the census was instituted about 1911, it seems increased, to their detriment, to 14,000.

Their occupation has been and is agricultural, but to this they added, before coming under the British suzerainty, a little banditry. They were not cruel; indeed, they seem to have regarded the looting of fat Turkis on their way to Mecca or the Khergiz of the Pamirs in part as a sport. But it was a sport that often ended in failure and a long journey home without food.

As brigands they showed their wonderful powers of endurance, travelling for miles along cruel precipices and crossing turbulent rivers at a speed none other could accomplish. They were, of course, much feared, and in 1891, Colonel Durand led an expedition to stop their practices. It seems that they were not unwilling to stop. Durand (*The Making of a Frontier*, 1894) discovered that they did not care to neglect their fields for banditry. Agriculture was their real desire, and true agriculturists are not military. "As brigands," says Durand, "they appear to have acted always on the orders of their chief, and the admirable culture of their ground, the immense and persistent labour spent on their irrigation channels, and on the retaining walls of their terraced fields," showed him clearly where their interests as a people lay.

Since brigandage has had to be abandoned as an extra source of income by the chiefs, its place has been taken by the profit received from the hire of porterage by travellers and mountaineers. The Hunza are quite exceptional porters. All mountaineers are agreed on this point. Two quotations from Volume 71 (1928) of the Journal of the Royal Geographical Society are examples of the general testimony.

General Bruce, of Mount Everest fame, recounted in 1928 at the Royal Geographical Society, how, in 1894, he had to call up the one-time Hunza Rifles,; how they left their flocks away up in the mountains, collected their kit, and "went to Gilgit in one march of sixty-five miles of very bad country indeed. . . . I found the Hunza people most charming and perfectly companionable. They are as active as any people can possibly be . . . and as slab climbers nobody in the world can beat the Hunza men. For very hard work in the mountains, if we had a trained body, they would not prove inferior to our best Sherpa porters," who have so nobly assisted our Everest climbers almost to the top of the world, but not quite.

The second testimony is that of Captain C. Y. Morris, who explored the Hunza side valleys and glaciers in 1927. "These men were with us for just on two months," he said at the same meeting of the Royal Geographical Society in 1928. "During this time they were continuously on the move and over what is probably some of the worst country in the world for laden men. Always ready to turn their hand to anything, they were, I think, the most cheerful and willing set of men with whom I have ever travelled. . . . At the worse part of all we halted in order to help the porters across. They disdained our proffered assistance, however, and came over, climbing like cats, and with never a murmur at the hardships of this day's work."

If there is anything to try the nerves in these parts and give the equivalent of neurasthenia, it must be the danger and the exhausting work of porterage. Other porters give up, as the readers of the tales of recent expeditions, such as that which conquered Nanda Devi, know. Not so the Hunza. They know neither the fear nor the weariness which spoils the will.

Far from being nervous or morose, nearly every visitor testifies to their freedom from quarrels and exceptional cheerfulness. This cheerfulness, one notes, seems to be a characteristic of the little Tibetans of Baltistan, Tibetans, Chinese, Koreans, and Japanese, all of whom, we shall see, follow certain similar principles of agriculture.

The Hunza originally were brought into contact with the British power owing to their interference with trade, which was by the same British converted from a hindrance to an assistance. But no people, of course, can exist upon banditry or porterage. "Far from being mere robber tribes," wrote Biddulph in 1880, of the Hunza, "they are settled agricultural communities."

Here also, as might be expected, they excel. They are admirable cultivators, far famed as such and "conspicuously ahead of all their neighbours in brain and sinew," stated

Schomberg. Their big irrigation conduit, the Berber, is "famous everywhere in Central Asia."

They are also what really follows from being capable agriculturists, namely, good craftsmen. Amongst the peoples of the Agency not only are they "as tillers of the soil quite in a class apart," writes Schomberg, "they alone—and this always strikes me as truly remarkable—are good craftsmen. As carpenters and masons, as gunsmiths, ironworkers, or even as goldsmiths, as engineers for roads, bridges or canals, the Hunza men are outstanding."

Lastly, as Mr. C. P. Skrine notes in *Chinese Central Asia* (1926), as dancers "they are incomparably finer than the well-known Cuttack dancing of the North-west Frontier."

As to food, owing to their excellent agriculture they have enough to eat, except the few weeks preceding the summer harvest. They have wheaten bread, barley and millet, a variety of vegetables and fruits. They have milk, buttermilk, clarified butter, and curd-cheese. They have occasional meat. They rarely have any fish or game. They take wine, mostly about the time of Christmas. They used to make spirits, but that has been forbidden.

It is important to note, as has been already stated, that since the suzerainty of the British the population has, it seems, increased, a common phenomenon when such a people comes in contact with the west. There is, therefore, less food for them than in the past, and Colonel D. L. Lorimer, who was Political Agent at Gilgit 1920-4, and revisited the Hunza and lived amongst them at Aliabad, 1933-4, four miles from the capital, Baltit, told me that not only did they seem smaller to him at his second visit, but that the children appeared under-nourished for the weeks preceding the first summer harvests half way through June; and, moreover, that the children suffered at that time of year from impetigo, or sores of the skin, all of which vanished when the more abundant food came. The supply of land and water is not to-day sufficient for the people at the pre-harvest period, the climate of Hunza being arid.

The most conspicuous feature of the Hunza diet is the large quantity of fruit they eat, fresh in the summer and at other times dried, either alone or in wheaten cakes. There is so much fruit in Hunza that "even the animals," said Durand, "take the fruit diet, and you see donkeys, cows and goats eating the fallen mulberries. The very dogs feed on them, and our fox-terriers took to the fruit regimen most kindly and became quite connoisseurs."

The daily eating is given by Schomberg as: nothing before going out in the early morning to the fields; after two or three hours of work, bread, pulses and vegetables with milk; at mid-day, fresh fruit or dried apricots kneaded with water; in the evening these same foods, with meat on rare occasions.

This food seems simple and primitive. It will be found, on amplification, that it is neither simple nor is it primitive in the sense of being crude, and the full understanding of it will not be reached until almost the last pages of this book.

The Hunza are Moslems, but they do not confine their women, who go about freely. Nor do they refrain from wine. On the contrary, they grow good grapes and enjoy home-made wine. They, and the people of Punyal, indeed, shock the more orthodox Moslems in those parts by their fondness for public jollifications. The Mir, or ruler, treats his visitors to his home-brew and they find it sound and comforting. Bruce suggested to his fellow-geographers that this wine is one of the causes of the great cheeriness of the Hunza.

Their life is one of the open air, of course, for men, women and children work in the fields. But they have to face the cold and storms of winter. The Hunza houses are often three storeys high and are better built and more light and airy than elsewhere in the Gilgit Agency. Moreover, owing to a shortage of fuel or a liking for better air, the Hunza, though they spend much time indoors during the stormy time of winter, do not fill the main living-room of the house with the dense smoky atmosphere which Durand speaks of as horrible in the houses of the Hindu-Kush generally in mid-winter.

As regards the disposal of human excreta, the Hunza here, as in other matters of great importance, follow the same principles as the Tibetans and Chinese. They pass their excreta into hidden privies, as do their Tibetan neighbours in

Baltistan. From time to time these privies are opened and the material is added to the compost, which they use for the manuring of the soil.

Their water they keep in closed, separate cisterns, so that their animals cannot drink from them. Open water tanks are provided for their beasts.

So the Hunza houses are better than their neighbours, their water is separate and protected, and their sanitation has the time-honoured approval of the Far East. Here, in these matters of ventilation, water-supply, and sanitation, they also show superiority; but, especially in winter ventilation, not such as can well account for the superiority of their physique. Something these better ways may well contribute, but not enough to give a full and sufficient reason.

Schomberg, therefore, asks the question : "Can it be race?" He gives many pages to answering the question.

As the first settlement of Nagir was from Hunza, the Hunza and Nagiris have been classed as one race. But the first settlement was many centuries ago, and since then many Kashmiris have entered Nagir and overwhelmed the earlier settlers. But they were kept out of Hunza. About the only remnant of relationship between the two peoples is that they both speak the Burushaski tongue. So do some people in Yasin and Punyal. There has been mixture. This is even seen in Hunza. But the majority of the Hunza in Hunza are distinguished by their fair skins, and they themselves scoff at being of the same blood as the smaller, dark Nagiris.

"Still less," says Schomberg, "are the Hunza folk of the same stock as those of the rest of the Indus valley. It is certainly difficult to understand how anyone, after having dealings with the Hunza people, could imagine that they had anything in common with their neighbours of Nagir, still less with the inhabitants of Gilgit or the Indus valley."

Their very language is a peculiar and difficult tongue, Burushaski, only spoken in Hunza and parts of Nagir, and a little in Punyal, whose men Schomberg, as already quoted, places as second to the Hunza. Sir Aurel Stein says something very significant about Burushaski in *Sand buried Ruins of*

Khotan (1906). It has "no apparent connection with either the Indian or the Iranian family of languages, and seems an erratic block left here by some bygone wave of conquest. . . . How the small race which speaks the language of Hunza has come to occupy these valleys will perhaps never be cleared up by historical evidence. But its preservation between the Dards on the south and the Iranians and Turki tribes on the north is clearly due to the isolated position of the country."

The Hunza people become now mysterious, as well as men of unequalled physique and health. They are something very old, an erratic block of an ancient world, still perhaps with its peculiar knowledge and traditions, and preserved in that profound cleft of theirs from the decay of time.

The ruling families of Hunza people make a claim to being descended from the soldiers of Alexander or even from Alexander himself, much as English families like to say their ancestors came over with the Conqueror. High-flown though this may seem, still there is one thing a little strange.

The Hunza, as Moslems, will not be photographed stripped. That is an unforgivable affront. Yet there is one such photo extant. It shows a man of medium height, broad shoulders, full chest, wide costal arch, narrow waist, small belly and strong legs. If one looks at this photo and then at the Æginetan Sculptures lodged in the Glyptothek of Munich, one sees rare men of peculiar deep-chested breathing, feeding efficiency and powerful motility. Most strangely and unexpectedly these sculptured men and the photoed Hunza appear the same. The photo might be the statues and the statues the photo.

Schomberg calls this claim of descent from the great Conqueror fantastic, and so it is, and any speculation with present knowledge upon a possible marvellous nest of pure-bred preservation of the classic Greek is equally fantastic. All one can say is that this people of Hunza, so unique amongst peoples, is no less unique in its racial characters. Everything suggests that in its remoteness it may preserve from the distant past, things that the modern world has forgotten and does not any longer understand. And amongst those things are perfect physique and health.

Chapter II

A REVOLUTION IN OUTLOOK

ROBERT McCARRISON, now Major-General Sir Robert McCarrison, qualified as a medical practitioner at Queen's University, Belfast, in 1900. He entered the Indian Medical Service and sailed for India on his twenty-third birthday.

He was posted as regimental medical officer to the Indian troops, stationed as warden to the frontier march of Chitral, between the Gilgit Agency on the east and Afghanistan on the west, in the heart of a country which, as we shall see in the penultimate chapter, is likely to prove one of the utmost significance in the history of food.

McCarrison had the inborn mind of a research worker. He quickly displayed it in the accustomed manner of medical research. Eighteen months after his arrival in India he was stationed at the isolated Fort of Drosh. The winter was cold but healthy. In the summer it was hot and dry, and then, as he reports in his Lloyd Roberts Lecture in 1937, "there fell upon us a strange sickness which few escaped." Here was the characteristic opportunity of the young medical research worker—a strange sickness.

McCarrison seized the opportunity with unalloyed scientific gladness, for the disease was not a serious one—a sharp three day-fever. He made every sort of investigation possible with his meagre equipment. He observed and tabulated the outbreak of the epidemic, the nature of its spread, the ages of the sufferers, its great prevalence amongst new-comers, the immunity of those previously attacked, and its absence above a certain altitude. He sent for his microscope and some simple laboratory apparatus. He examined hundreds of blood films for malaria and found it absent. Quinine also had no effect on the fever or its symptoms. He tried to grow microbes from the blood of patients and failed. He inoculated volunteers with the blood of the affected with no result. He made mosquito surveys and sand-fly surveys, to see if the fever was possibly conveyed by their bites. He finally came strongly to suspect sand-flies as the conveyers of the disease, and again and again submitted volunteers to bites by these insects, which had been fed on fevered patients, and again with no result. So he published his results without proving the cause, and "Three-day Fever of Chitral" figured in the text-books. Soon it was recognised that this fever prevailed, as McCarrison predicted, in other parts of India, and also in Dalmatia, Malta, Crete, and other Mediterranean stations. In 1908 Doerr confirmed McCarrison's suspicions, and the disease henceforth came to be known as sand-fly fever.

The young McCarrison followed this excellent piece of research with one which still claims his interest, though that interest has now merged into the greater one of his later work.

In his Milroy Lectures of 1912 he described what the research worker, working by means of the outlook of disease, regards as a piece of good fortune. In the Gilgit Agency, to which he was appointed surgeon 1904-1911, another experiment on a grand scale in disease, not health, was being carried out by nature, in a manner that excited his keen interest. The disease was that of goitre, or enlargement of the thyroid gland, which lies in front of the wind-pipe.

In the introduction of his first lecture he expressed his joy in being provided with a suitable subject for his abilities in these words: "Having the good fortune to reside for some ten years in a part of India where goitre and cretinism prevail with great intensity, and which is probably one of the purest regions of endemic goitre in the world, I have had exceptional opportunities for carrying out extensive observations and experiments, not only on animals, but on man also." He then went on to describe his researches to date. Needless to say they were thorough and profitable. They were based on the disease as exhibited particularly in the nine villages which are collectively known as Gilgit, where he himself was stationed. He succeeded so well in his research that he was eventually able to give himself and fifteen volunteers the local disease and then to cure it. There's no need to go into the course of these researches, interesting and illuminating though they are. The chief effect, from the point of view of this book, is that they led to McCarrison being relieved of the routine duties of a medical officer and separated as a research worker. In 1913 he was transferred to the Central Institute, Kasauli, with its well-equipped laboratories, to pursue his investigations with all the advantages which well-equipped laboratories, scientific colleagues and literature offer.

In 1912 Sir Gowland Hopkins had made public his work on accessory food factors, to which Casimir Funk a year later gave the name of vitamins. McCarrison, reading the work, at once thought that maybe a very important clue to the enigma of goitre lay in a deficiency of vitamins in the food which goitrous people eat. So he began experiments in the Kasauli laboratory designed to give pigeons goitre. He fed them on diets defective in vitamins. Something different happened. The birds did not develop goitre, but some of them, as was expected, developed a disease called polyneuritis. Then it was found that these birds were overrun by specific microbes. Now came the surprise. Some of the healthy birds, the stock of the laboratory who were well fed before any experiments were tried upon them, also harboured these microbes, but they were not ill. The ill-fed birds, on the other hand, were mortally sick. If, however, the healthy birds were fed on the food defective in vitamins, they too got the polyneuritis and died. Good feeding, it seemed, protected the birds against the microbes, but faulty feeding led to a microbic triumph. Thus was McCarrison brought into a field of "deficiency diseases," that is to say, diseases due definitely to faulty food. Then came the War, and nothing more was done in research until 1918.

Now, it must be carefully noted that up to this time McCarrison's research work, brilliant though it was, ran on the conventional medical lines. It was concerned with certain diseases and it had the outlook of disease—such is the cause of Chitral three-day fever, such are the causes of goitre, of cretinism, of pigeon's polyneuritis, and so on. There was no revolution of outlook as yet.

In 1918 McCarrison returned to research under the Research

Fund Association of India. He took up the study of deficiency diseases, which had first excited his interest, as a side issue of his work at Kasauli on goitre. In 1921 he published a book entitled *Studies in Deficiency Diseases*.

Now studies in deficiency diseases clearly entail for contrast the picture, if not the study, of efficient animals. Animals or birds, which are kept for experiments, are kept in ordinary health by hygienic care, and sound food. They are, for this reason, known as controls, for it is by comparison of their condition with that of their experimented comrades that the effect of any experimental testing can be observed.

It was when his mind was dwelling on the healthy that the picture of the people of Hunza returned to McCarrison.

When he was Agency Surgeon at Gilgit, the Hunza, though sixty miles away, were his official patients. Like other Europeans who met them, he was greatly impressed by their fine physique, but his research-brain was busy on illness, goitre and cretinism in particular, and these illnesses, like most others, the Hunza failed to get. As a people they offered very poor fare to a researching physician.

The ultimate objects of McCarrison's experiments on faultily fed animals were, of course, human. They were to find out what and to what degree diseases in Indian peoples were caused by faulty food. So the memory of the Hunza came back to McCarrison with peculiar vividness. They had no such diseases. They came before McCarrison as a picture of the high attainment man can reach in health and physique.

"My own experience," he wrote in his book, "provides an example of a race unsurpassed in perfection of physique and in freedom from disease in general. I refer to the people of the State of Hunza, situated in the extreme northernmost point of India. . . . Amongst these people the span of life is extraordinarily long; and such service as I was able to render them during the seven years I spent in their midst was confined chiefly to the treatment of accidental lesions, the removal of senile cataract, plastic operations for granular lids, or the treatment of maladies wholly unconnected with food supply."

There were two diseases of the eyes, cataract in old people

and irritation of the inner lining of the lids. If the winter ventilation of the living-rooms in Hunza had been better, even though not so foul as that of most houses in the Hindu-Kush, which, Durand wrote, choked the unfortunate inhabitants, these two diseases might also have been excluded.

In his Mellon Lecture, delivered at Pittsburgh, in the U.S.A., in 1922, on "Faulty Food in Relation to Gastro-Intestinal Disorder," this people of the remote Himalayas, whose name he did not give to his American audience, but undoubtedly the Hunza and such allied people as the Punyalis, again presented themselves to him—almost as control human beings in the vast laboratory of nature, in which civilised people, and especially Americans, were very prone to gastro-intestinal disorders.

"During the period of my association with these people," he said, "I never saw a case of asthenic dyspepsia, of gastric or duodenal ulcer, of appendicitis, of mucous colitis, of cancer. . . . Among these people the 'abdomen over-sensitive' to nerve impressions, to fatigue, anxiety or cold was unknown. The consciousness of the existence of this part of their anatomy was, as a rule, related solely to the feeling of hunger. Indeed, their buoyant abdominal health has, since my return to the west, provided a remarkable contrast with the dyspeptic and colonic lamentations of our highly civilized communities."

So the picture of a healthy people in 1921-2 strongly coloured McCarrison's thought.

His work on deficiency diseases was, as has been said, to discover their prevalence in India. One aspect of this study had been of peculiar importance to the Government, namely the prevalence of the diseases amongst the native troops during the War. The Government had to be informed what foods their soldiers should take to avoid these diseases, if possible, in future campaigns.

This, fortunately, brought McCarrison into research contact with the fighting races of India—Punjabis, Dogras, Rajputs, Brahmins, Jats, Ghoorkas, Pathans, and Sikhs. It did not, however, bring any Hunza men again under his observation, for, though there had at one time been the Hunza Rifles, to whose marching powers Bruce testified in our first chapter, they were soon disbanded, and further enlistment of the Hunza in any form prohibited, owing to the strong objection of the Mir to his subjects leaving the country.

Of these fighting men, McCarrison selected the Pathans and Sikhs as men of exceptional physique. He grouped them in his mind and writing henceforth with the Hunza, though he always gave the Hunza the premier place. A brief account of these two fighting peoples is therefore necessary.

Looking at a map of Afghanistan, one sees that its north-eastern corner projects a long thin tongue to the east. This forms a northern cap to Chitral and the Gilgit Agency, and its tip touches the Hunza river cleft.

Near Chitral town the eastern border of Afghanistan turns sharply south. Between it and the plains of the Punjab are the North-west Frontier Provinces. This is the country of the Pathans.

The Pathans, therefore, are not the immediate neighbours of the Hunza, nor are they allied to them in race. The Pathans are in part Semitic, their neighbours, the Afghans, being yet more Semitic. The Pathans call themselves Beni-Israel, as descendants of the ten lost tribes of Israel.

But they are like the people of Hunza in that they are great hillsmen, though their mountains are not so vast. But in their life as hillsmen-agriculturalists, they form a group with the hillsmen of Eastern Afghanistan, of Chitral and of the Gilgit Agency. The significance of this will be seen in the penultimate chapter upon the Hunza Foods.

There are about a million Pathans. They are a very vigorous people. Here is an account of the famous Afridi Pathans, who live in the neighbourhood of the Khyber Pass: "The Afridi, in appearance, is generally a fine, tall athletic highlander, whose springy step, even in traversing the dirty streets of Peshawur, at once denotes his mountain origin." His appearance immediately prejudices Englishmen in his favour and "there are few brought into contact with him who do not at least begin with an enthusiastic admiration of his manliness."

The Sikhs are not hillsmen, but belong to the river plains of the Punjab. They are a religious, not a racial community. The greater number of them are converted Jats. They are an independent people and admirable agriculturists. "In agriculture," wrote Captain Bingley, *The Sikhs* (1899), "the Jat-Sikh is pre-eminent. No one can rival him as a landowner or yeoman cultivator. He calls himself a *Zamindar*, or husbandman, as often as a Jat, and his women and children work with him in the fields. Indeed, it is a common saying in the Punjab that the Jat's baby has a ploughshare for a plaything."

The Sikh is up at dawn and at work in his field, taking a little food left over from the previous day before he leaves his home. About midday, when the sun gets powerful, his women bring him out a substantial meal of coarse ground wheaten *chapattis* smeared with butter, porridges of grains and pulses, vegetables, and when in season, raw, green gram or *sarson*. He washes all this down with copious draughts of spiced buttermilk, which he calls *lassi*. He takes a further substantial meal of similar foods at the end of the day's work. He eats sprouting gram. He eats fruit, though he cannot get the abundance of it which Hunza and Pathans get. He takes meat sparingly, sometimes freely.

He works hard, but he is spared the necessitous exercise which the mountains force upon the Hunza and Pathan. Nevertheless, he likes extra exercise in the way of sports and games. He is fond of running and jumping, lifting and tossing weights, throwing quoits, or weilding huge wooden clubs. When young he is fond of wrestling. But, as Bingley observed, the Jat-Sikh is usually too much occupied with agricultural labour to spare much time for games.

Such were the pick of the fighting men of India whom McCarrison associated with the Hunza in the perfection of their physique. "The Sikhs, the Pathans, and certain Himalaya tribes, than whom it would be difficult to find races, whether in the east or west, of finer physical development, hardihood and powers of endurance," he wrote in an article in *The Practitioner* in 1925, and then gave the premier place to the Hunza: "These people are unsurpassed by any Indian race in perfection of physique; they are long-lived, vigorous in youth and age, capable of great endurance and enjoy a remarkable freedom from disease in genaral."

It is clear in this article of 1925 upon "The Relationship of Diet to the Physical Efficiency of Indian Races" that McCarrison's review of the fighting races had removed him from the conventional attitude of medical research to an over-riding interest in healthy peoples. The question that now pre-sented itself to his mind was : "How is it that man can be such a magnificent physical creature as the Hunza, the Sikh, or the Pathan ?"

Health is wholeness. The careful reader of McCarrison's *Studies in Deficiency Diseases* will note that wholeness lay in the very texture of his mind. The work reveals an intellectual passion for wholeness. Up to that time, as he himself later pointed out in the Lloyd Roberts Lecture, research workers in malnutrition had studied the effects of faulty food upon the nerves, the eyes, the bones and so on. They fragmented the subject. He was the first "to survey the whole realm of the body by microscopic means." He had to see wholly. One can, indeed, watch this sense of wholeness increasing in his work, until it shaped itself in the whole view of health which will be presented in the last chapter.

So when he had to study the Sikh, Pathan, and others, he seemed to step into what was really quite a new atmosphere of observation. His approach to it was long, but it led him no less surely to a new outlook than did the tracks which brought stout Cortez upon a peak of Darien. McCarrison is now impressed and absorbed by certain people's efficiency, with deficiency only as a background and contrast; by health as a whole thing, and not the medical health, namely, the state which is reached by recovery from a disease. The pyramid of medical art, built up of innumerable studies of an increasing number of diseases, was turned upon its top, and, as a new position, in precarious stability. But McCarrison managed to sustain it, and from the small apex formed by Hunza, Sikh and Pathan physique and health, he proceeded to view the ills of both civilized and uncivilized man.

This was a complete reversal of the accustomed outlook of medical research. We have all become so weary of revolutions in these days that I fear the very phrase "a revolution of medical thought" may be objectionable. But that is what this was. The old traditional way of thought, namely, from separate diseases or groups of diseases to the recovery of average health, was displaced by looking from the healthiest procurable peoples to the innumerable ailments and diseases of men. It was in the strictest sense of the word a revolution, a turning round.

The right-about is the unique character of McCarrison's later research work. It is this which separates it from his earlier research work. Of course, one cannot always draw a mark, as one can across a race track and say: "Here is the start." One could collect many instances of tentative approaches to this change of direction in the work of others as well as that of McCarrison. Every revolution has such presages. But in McCarrison's work this conversion was complete, except for an occasional relapse to the subject of goitre. From this time his work starts from these men of unsurpassed physique, and is an enquiry as to what it was that gave them bodily excellence in such full measure.

Chapter III

THE TRANSFERENCE TO EXPERIMENTAL
SCIENCE

In 1927 McCarrison was appointed Director of Nutrition Research in India under the Research Fund Association. He was not only director, he was, as he told the members of the Royal Commission on Agriculture in India, the only officer engaged on work on nutrition, so he had, as it were, only to direct himself. He was given a laboratory and headquarters at Coonoor, upon the beautiful Nilgiri plateau of the Madras Presidency, and there he directed his work and that of his excellent Indian assistants to the transference of the health of Hunza, Sikh and Pathan to experimental science.

For this work McCarrison chose albino rates. Rats are largely used in nutritional laboratories. They offer many advantages for experimental work on foods. They are omnivorous and they like practically all human food. They are small animals, and therefore cheap to feed; they breed readily in captivity, and their span of life is short, so that their whole life history can be watched.

The first object of McCarrison was to see if the rats in their small sphere of life could be made exceptional rats in physique and health. He put them in good conditions of air, sunlight, and cleanliness, and he chose as a diet for them one based on those of the three people of excellent physique, the Hunza, the Pathan, and the Sikhs.

He did not, however, give the full diet of any of these peoples in one particular, that of fruit. The Hunza eat fresh and dried fruit abundantly. The Pathans are also large eaters of fruits. The Sikhs, with a climate less suitable to fruit, eat less than the Hunza and Pathan. They cannot be distinguished as great fruit eaters. The rats were given no fruit. The foods they received were those of these peoples of north-western India minus fruit.

The diet given to the rats was chapattis, or flat bread, made of wholemeal wheat flour, lightly smeared with fresh butter, sprouted pulse, fresh raw carrots and fresh raw cabbage *ad libitum*, unboiled whole milk, a small ration of meat with bones once a week, and an abundance of water, both for drinking and washing.

In this experiment 1,189 rats were watched from birth to the twenty-seventh month, an age in the rat which corresponds to that of about fifty-five years in man. The rats were killed and carefully examined at all ages up to the twenty-seventh month of life by naked-eye post-mortem examination.

The result was very remarkable. Disease was abolished. This astonishing consequence, however, must be given in McCarrison's own words in the first of two lectures given at the College of Surgeons in 1931.

"During the past two and a quarter years there has been no case of illness in this 'universe' of albino rats, no death from natural causes in the adult stock, and, but for a few accidental deaths, no infantile mortality. Both clinically and at post-mortem examination this stock has been shown to be remarkably free from disease. It may be that some of them have cryptic disease of one kind or another, but, if so, I have failed to find either clinical or macroscopical evidence of it."

By putting the rats on a diet similar to that of certain peoples of Northern India, the rats became "hunzarised," that is they "enjoyed a remarkable freedom from disease," words used by McCarrison in 1925 of the Hunza. They even went further. Except for an occasional tape worm cyst they had no visible disease at all.

Now, the reader might think that a statement that any small "universe" had been freed from disease would have created a profound impression amongst medical men. It did not do so, any more than Lister's announcement of the first results of antiseptic surgery created any stir. In Lister's days surgeons were so accustomed to pus and blood poisoning, they could not think in terms of a surgery without them. Similarly, medical men are so accustomed to a great number of diseases, they cannot think of any small "universe" without disease. In all revolutions this is the case. It is the established profession, or class or aristocracy, which finds it most difficult to think in terms of the change.

This is very noticeable in the professional comments of that time upon McCarrison's lectures. Actually they were very meagre. I only found one reference in the corresponding columns of the leading journals of the few weeks following the lectures. The British Medical Journal itself did, however, devote a leading article. This article treated McCarrison's work purely from the point of view of diseases which diet would prevent or help to prevent. It overlooked the astonishing relation of a remarkable health of human groups being transferred to rats as a perfect health.

"We are passing from a period in which bacteria were held of more surgical importance than diet to one in which a knowledge of diet is to be regarded as more important than a knowledge of bacteria. It is the physician or dietitian who is leading the way. Who would have thought ten years ago that an error in diet would render us liable to such diverse conditions as middle-ear disease, duodenal ulcer, renal calculus or cystitis?" One notes it is liability to diseases, not remarkable health, that is the underlying philosophy.

It is in one sense, nevertheless, fair comment on the lectures themselves. Being prepared especially for surgeons, they were given a surgical setting, and were, therefore, gathered around a number of surgical diseases. It was indeed this familiar setting which caused the unfamiliar significance of the transfer of the remarkable health of certain humans to the rats to be dimmed. This was the light which should have shone forth amidst the familiar murk of human illness. This was the positive meaning, the health or whole meaning of the experiment.

The health was transferred by foods. It was not, as we shall see, transferred by any particular hygienic methods common to the Hunza and the rats. In air, light, etc., there were some resemblances, but in scientific hygiene that of the rats was superior.

First, as regards climate, Coonoor stands 6,000 feet high and Hunza is nearly 8,000 feet high. Coonoor is on a tableland and its climate is equable, the annual range of temperature being from 50 degrees to 80 degrees Fahr. It has not that hard, cold winter of Hunza, in which for two months, having little to do outside, the people spend their time in stuffy rooms. The rats in their roomy cages got plenty of air and sunlight all the year round.

So in the matter of domestic ventilation, the rats were better off than the humans. It was the humans who in winter were wont to live in atmospheres like those of rat-holes.

The Hunza have no fear abroad or at home, but rats are timid when living in airy cages and sunlight and unable to hide. So, to avoid fear and its bad effect on health, the rats were screened from observation and their attendants were trained to attend upon them without alarming them.

Their cages were hosed out once a day, they were daily put in the sun, and they were lined daily with clean straw. The test of cleanliness was that no smell at all could be detected in the room where the cages were kept. It cannot be said that, in spite of different habits, the Hunza houses were more hygienic than this. The balance here lies with the rats.

In natural exercise and in adventure in getting the means of life the rats were restricted. The cages were large enough for the animals to move about in their slow cautious way, with little darts forward, but not for the hot scamper of danger, which calls upon the supremest physical qualities, such as the Hunza show as cragsmen in perilous places. Here the fortune lay with Hunza or rat, according as one values adventure or safety first as a factor of health.

These additional "environmental conditions: cleanliness and comfort," as McCarrison calls them, were not, therefore, common to rat and Hunza. An exact imitation of Hunza or Pathan conditions was not possible in these particulars. They were, therefore, so arranged that they were good and constant. They were kept the same for all the rats in all McCarrison's experiments. Then, if one batch of rats with one diet kept well and another with another diet got ill, the conclusion that the diet in the second case was faulty was obvious. This is a common method of experimental science.

The only thing, therefore, that was common to rat and man in this first experiment was the diet. Here in the great cleft of Hunza was a little oasis of a few thousand beings of almost perfect health, and here in the cages of Coonoor was a little oasis of a thousand and more albino rats also in perfect health. The only link connection between these two otherwise dissimilar sets of living things was a similar kind of diet.

McCarrison now linked up other batches of rats in the same constant conditions of cleanliness and comfort with other peoples of India by their diets. He was in a most enviable position for trying out diets as a whole. The Indian subcontinent provides so many different races and different habits and diets. Hence McCarrison was able to sit in his sanctum at Coonoor and connect up his rats with teeming peoples near and far, and in the mirror of the rats read the dietetic fates of the peoples.

He took the customary diets of the poorer peoples of Bengal and Madras, consisting of rice, pulses, vegetables, condiments, perhaps a little milk. He gave these to rats.

Now, this diet immediately opened the lid of Pandora's box for the rats of Coonoor, and diseases and miseries of many kinds flew forth.

McCarrison made a list of them as found by him in 2,243 rats fed on faulty Indian diets. Here it is as given by him at the Royal College of Surgeons in, necessarily, technical language: "Lung diseases: pneumonia, broncho-pneumonia, bronchiectasis, pyothorax, pleurisy, hæmothorax.

"Diseases of the nose and accessory sinuses: sinusitis.

"Diseases of the ear: otitis media or pus in the middle ear.

"Diseases of the upper respiratory passages: adenoid growths.

"Diseases of the eye: conjunctivitis, corneal ulceration, keratomalacia, panophthalmitis.

"Gastro-intestinal diseases: dilated stomach, gastric ulcer, epithelial new growths in the stomach, cancer of the stomach (in two cases only), duodenitis, enteritis, gastro-intestinal dystrophy, stasis.

"Diseases of the urinary tract : pyonephrosis, hydronephrosis, pyelitis, renal calculus, ureteral calculus, dilated ureters, vesical calculus, cystitis, incrusted cystitis.

"Diseases of the reproductive system : inflammation of the uterus, ovaritis, death of the fœtus *in utero,* premature birth, uterine hæmorrhage, hydrops testis.

"Diseases of the skin : loss of hair, dermatitis, abscesses, gangrene of the tail, gangrene of the feet, subcutaneous œdema.

"Diseases of the blood : anæmia, a 'pernicious' type of anæmia, *Bartonella Muris* anæmia.

"Diseases of the lymph and other glands : cysts in the sub-maxillary glands and accessory glands in the base of the tongue, abscesses in the same, and occasionally also in the inguinal glands, enlarged adrenal glands, atrophy of the thymus, enlarged mesenteric, bronchial and other lymph glands.

"Diseases of the endocrine system : lymph-adenoid goitre, and, very occasionally, hæmorrhage into the pancreas.

"Diseases of the nervous system : polyneuritis.

"Diseases of the heart : cardiac atrophy, occasionally cardiac hypertrophy, myocarditis, pericarditis, and hydro-pericardium.

"Oedema."

That is the complete list. Freeing it of its technical dressing, in plain English it means that the rats, which were fed on the diets eaten by millions of Indians of Bengal and Madras, got diseases of every organ they possessed, namely eyes, noses, ears, lungs, hearts, stomachs, intestines, kidneys, bladders, reproductive organs, blood, ordinary glands, special glands, and nerves. The liver and the brain, it may be noted, do not occur in the list. The liver was as a fact found to be diseased in conjunction with the diseases of the gastro-intestinal tract. The examination of the brain requires a care-ful opening of the small bony brain case of the rat and adds greatly to the time needed for post-mortem examinations.

This list denotes a pretty comprehensive lot of troubles to

be loaded on to simple little creatures like rats as a result of eating faulty Indian diets. In a list given five years later in the Cantor Lectures, McCarrison adds a few further diseases, such as general weakness, lassitude, irritability, loss of hair, ulcers, boils, bad teeth, crooked spines, distorted vertebræ, and so on.

Considering again the simplicity of the rat and its limitation in things human, the list is, comparatively speaking, almost as complete as the list of contents of a stately text-book of medicine. The diseases of the mind and other very special diseases are omitted. One cannot exactly diagnose neurasthenia, hysteria, and schizophrenia, in the rat.

Yet even in rats conditions like to these arise from faulty diet. For example, in later experiment, McCarrison gave a set of rats the diet of the poorer classes of England; white bread, margarine, sweetened tea, boiled vegetables, tinned meats and jams of the cheaper sort. On this diet, not only did the rats grow badly, but they developed what one might call rat-neurasthenia, and more than neurasthenia. "They were nervous and apt to bite their attendants; they lived unhappily together, and by the sixteenth day of the experiment they began to kill and eat the weaker ones amongst them."

We can add neurasthenia and ferocity to weaker brethren to the list.

We are left then at the end of these experiments with two vividly contrasted sets of little animals in this small "universe" of Coonoor—those on good and those on faulty diet; the healthy and the sickly; and certain mental characters, in contrast, the good tempered and live-and-let-live on the one hand, the bad-tempered and cannibalistic on the other.

And it must be carefully noted that in the case of the healthy rats, the diet was a whole thing. Not only was it their diet from weaning to death, but their mothers were "stock" rats, that is to say, they were being fed on the diet of certain peoples of north-western India, when their off-spring were conceived, when they were carrying them, and when they were giving them the breast. The importance of this will be seen in the next chapter.

Chapter IV

THE START

WHEN should one begin a diet? That is an important question.

The sort of answer that has a wide appeal is: "You can carry on till forty. Then you should think of being careful about your food," or the practical individual answer: "Wait till you get indigestion."

The real answer to the question is that one should not oneself have to start a diet. It ought to be there as the Hunza diet is there. One ought to step into it as one steps into existence. One ought to get its benefits as one gets the benefits of air. One ought not to have indigestion, but be like the Hunza, only conscious of one's abdomen through the sensation of hunger. As to care after forty, the Hunza are vigorous in age as they are in youth. So it was that Mr. Skrine saw the Mir of Hunza at polo when nearly seventy. As captain of his side, after a goal, he had to gallop at full speed half-way up the ground, fling the ball into the air and smite it towards the opposing goal. "I saw the Mir, who in spite of his years is still a wonderful player, perform this feat, known as the *tambok*, eight times in succession and never once did he hit the ball less than a hundred yards."

So the answer to the question "When to start a diet?" is that one should be in it from the start. It should be there at conception, as the air is at birth.

Practically, in western urban civilisation this is not so. No one can rely on his abdominal organs and physique generally to that degree. We have got off the track and we have to get back to it, and how to do that, with the Hunza as a guide, will be shown in the last chapters. There also we will find pretty surprising things about starts.

Meanwhile, let us take the start here as individual, the conceiving of the individual in the environment of a right diet.

To do this, let us follow the great Lord Lister's favourite dictum: "Be strange to the familiar." We are all so accustomed to thinking of ourselves as Harry This or Beatrice That, that it is difficult for us to be strange to the familiar and remember that we were all once nameless microscopic specks.

It is as a microscopic speck that the individual life of a man, an animal, a fish, a tree, in fact any sort of life, starts. That is what we realise when we make ourselves strange to the familiar as regards the start. We don't start at birth.

There is the speck, ready to become a human being or fish or bird or tree. Each speck, therefore, is specific, but to each there is something common. The speck that is to become a human being becomes it through foods. The speck that is to become a fish becomes it through foods. The speck that is to become a tree becomes it through foods.

The specific qualities of each speck making one into a human being, another into a bird, belong to these great mysteries of being which we cannot penetrate and before which each, making himself strange to the familiar, must halt. It is then that we realise in the highest sense we *know* nothing, except that there is this mysterious power that can change these minute specks, apparently so familiar, into the immense diversity of living things.

So of specificity we can say nothing. But the development of each specific unit depends on one thing coming to it from the outer world, namely, food.

The human speck requires shelter, steady warmth, and the removal of waste products; the speck of a bird variable warmth and protection; the speck of a tree a fortunate security but no special provision of warmth. All of them require suitable food. Place the speck in arctic cold or torrid heat, on alpine heights or ocean's floor, let it be air-borne or buried in the soil, in each the speck shares the common factor of food.

So, making ourselves strange to the familiar, we might say: "At the start I was dependent for my health, not on physical exercise, the clean winds of the countryside, Viyella vests, stout boots, a touch of Kruschen in the morning, a good conscience and the approval of my neighbours, but on food. Food is primary."

What is primary remains primary.

At the start, then, the all-important thing for health is the foods (of which oxygen is then an unseparated part) which are brought by the mother's blood.

A healthy mother, eating healthy foods, is then a prerequisite for the good start. The rule, however, of the quite healthy mother is not absolute, for, if there happens to be a deficiency in her diet, it is she who suffers, not the child. If, for example, there is not sufficient calcium and iron for the pregnant woman and her foetus in her food, it is the growing life that seizes its full complement and the mother who gets pale and weak through deprivation.

Generally speaking, it is unquestionably the healthy mother who gives the speck a good start. This good start the Hunza people get. They get it as an unquestionable birth-right or conception-right. And the good start is transferable by diet. The mother rats fed by McCarrison on the Hunza-Pathan-Sikh diet never aborted nor was there infantile death.

On the other hand, female rats, fed by McCarrison on the foods of the poor Bengali or Madrassi, foods comparable to "the poorer class Britisher's diet," sometimes failed to give their conceptions anything more than a start and a brief course. They sometimes only got as far as producing false starts. They got inflammation of the womb and ovaries, and this led to abortion or premature birth. Sometimes there was no start at all, and they died without delivering themselves of their offspring. "Often I have seen deficiently fed rats that die in pregnancy," said McCarrison in his lecture, "and often also rats that come to term only to die with five or six foetuses in the womb."

That faulty food led to no starts or false starts was not, of course, discovered, but emphasised by these experiments. As long ago as 1906 Mr. S. M. Babcock in the U.S.A. planned out his famous Wisconsin experiment. Three groups of cattle were fed on the complete ripe plants of wheat, maize, and oats. Chemically these corn plants produced the same diet. Was it really the same? The results were as a fact very different.

The cows fed on maize, which is the only one of the three grains of purely American origin, did well and their calves were normal. Those fed on oats did moderately well. The wheat-fed cows did badly. They became rough-coated and gaunt. They produced thin, undersized young two to four weeks too soon, and the young were either born dead or they died within a few hours. This does not mean that the whole wheat plant is bad food compared to the whole maize plant. It only means that for these cows the whole maize plant provided a diet and the wheat plant failed to do so, for it is clear that on it the race of these cattle would have died out. But as a food, that is to say, just a part of a diet, wheat may well be superior to maize.

There are hard indicators of the adequacy of the start and the mother's diet in the teeth. The teeth are formed whilst the fœtus is in the womb and are within the gums at birth. Either before or when they erupt they can be made to tell the story of maternal diet and the start.

In his book *Nutrition and Diseases* (1934), Sir Edward Mellanby records this story, based upon Lady Mellanby's admirable work on teeth, with experiments on those of dogs: "If two comparable bitches are fed, one (A) on a diet of high calcifying qualitites, the second (B) on a poor calcifying diet, the teeth of the offspring are affected in two ways:—

(1) The actual calcification of the teeth taking place *in utero* of the fœtuses of A is better than in the fœtuses of B.

(2) After birth, if the diets of the puppies of A and B respectively are low calcifying qualities, the teeth of A's offspring—the well-fed mother—stand up more effectively to the bad conditions and are better formed than those of B's offspring. In other words, it would appear that if once the mechanism of calcification gets a good start as the result of perfect conditions *in utero* (in the womb), it is more difficult to upset by subsequent bad conditions."

What's bred in the teeth appears through the gums. Teeth, then, may be taken as the most convenient indicators of whether the mother's blood carried sound food or not. Even if dietary conditions after birth are not good, they are still indicators, for if the mother was healthy, it is harder for subsequent bad conditions to upset the good foundation. So written, it seems a truism, which needs no scientific proof.

Now, if defective teeth or even imperfect fitting of the projections and indentations of the upper and lower rows are indicators of the start, how many of us can boast of a perfect start? Even Ministers of Health, who reassure us on the state of out national nutrition, would seldom dare to show their teeth in proof of it. Their tongues are safer advocates than their teeth.

There is really no need to prove the widespread defectiveness of civilized teeth. It is too well known. The statements and statistics naturally vary according to how strict is the measure, but they are all on the very large side. Thus a well-known American odontologist, that is to say a specialist in the proper alignment and fitting of upper and lower rows of teeth together, stated recently that he had never seen a perfect fit in the mouth of an American-born white child. That is one hundred per cent and one can't go beyond that.

The statement of the League of Nations Committee on *The Problem of Nutrition* (Interim Report, Volume I) summed up the evidence before them on caries, or the decay of the teeth only, not misfit, in these words: "As regards dental caries, the enquiries carried out in various European countries have shown it to be present in from fifty to ninety-five per cent of the children examined. In a recent enquiry undertaken in Norway, only 160 out of the 25,000 school-children examined possessed perfect sets of teeth. According to the English report mentioned above, out of 3,303,983 children examined in 1933, 2,263,135 needed dental treatment."

This is sufficient to show, what scarcely anyone will deny, that the perfect start is somehow missed in modern civilization. Some may say that it is not the start, but the conditions after birth that are faulty. The two cannot be divided. A people whose traditions give them the perfect start give them also the right conditions after birth.

The great need of the right start is being recognised by authority in a somewhat feeble way. That is not authority's fault, for authority in England certainly cannot effect a radical revolution with a magic wand, or any other immediate means. One cannot leap out of a swamp.

Under the auspices of the Ministry of Health an experiment was organised from the Selly Oak Hospital and the report issued in 1936. This experiment did not go back to the start, but was an attempt to feed nursing mothers so that their children got sounder teeth. It proved abortive owing to the difficulty of finding out how strictly the mothers really followed the diet, etc.

A similar defect in the mother as a scientific object and witness is likely to make abortive a second attempt on the part of the State to approach the subject of the better start. It is that of giving the mothers and prospective mothers of the poorer classes milk. Here it is hard to be sure that the all-too-human mothers drink all the milk and do not share it out with the family or give some to an ailing child.

It is really essential to ask, why such attempts are so feeble. Not only do they not go back deliberately to the start, but they ignore the very essence of a diet, that it is a whole and that is why it gives health, which is a word also meaning whole— whole, hale, holy, health. Giving additional milk is patch-work, useful patchwork, no doubt, but patchwork never-theless.

Why then is there this lack of conviction about nutrition, why the lack of will towards it?

The answer to that question cannot lightly be given. It is involved in a trans-valuation of values, since that time when the modern world broke away from agricultural values and traditions and set up urban, money-making values in their place. The civilization of urban dominance may be better than the old. That is not the question here at issue. But it has within it intrinsic dangers. That no one can deny. And one of these dangers is the ill-judgment, the subjective judgment, of those of ill-physique. We have to-day as many ill-balanced judgments as we have men of the poor start.

Let me give an illustration. A few years ago I attended a big medical meeting, such as are held annually in the Empire. I had come from a country of balanced poise and movement, and after I had listened a little to the learned experts and professors upon the subject of health I became more and more inattentive to their speech and more and more interested in their lack of physical balance. I found myself taking notes, not of the lectures, but of the lecturers. They showed a lack of spontaneously assumed poise when speaking. They would stand crooked, place a foot on a step, withdraw it again, twist their fingers, scratch their heads or eyebrows, twitch, or kink their mouths sideways. It was also noticeable that these evidences of ill-balance were more marked in the laboratory-workers than whose who came from the country. One, whose occupation, and no doubt liking, took him much into the open air of the country, throughout his address placed his straight body firmly on well-planted legs with complete nervous control. Incidentally, his speech seemed to me the most wholesome and spacious in regard to the subject of health. Later I found that he had had an exceptional start and childhood.

I take it that what these speakers denoted would be roughly characteristic of most of us under like circumstances of self-consciousness, in the lack of poise and easy movement, which are characters of perfect physique. And this might well be expected, for few of us have really had a perfect start.

We cannot recapture that start, and in realising its value we may well feel that as adults we have missed that glory of the body, that easy poise and movement, that serenity of mental and physical rightness, that sound nerve, which might have been ours. We can, with care and knowledge, improve ourselves, but certain limitations have been set upon us which cannot now be overcome. So much we know.

What is less known is that because, physically, we are not as we should or could be, our outlook on health is not whole. It is conditioned by this lower state of physique and health.

We have become accustomed to look from this lower state, and the level we see we call normal, though in reality it is low grade. It is not to be supposed, for instance, that any of the professors and experts whom I heard and watched speaking upon health regarded themselves as other than normal. I also am regarded as normal or perhaps extra healthy, but at no time could I have walked sixty miles at a stretch and back again as an ordinary thing to do. At no time could I have joined in that speedy, terrific dance which Skrine witnessed. So, I think, is it with nearly all of us.

One cannot leap from the mire. We shall take time to lay firm ground to the whole meaning of health again. But we can comprehend it. It is not only the good start and the good continuance. There is much more to it than that, as will be seen. But the good start is one of its essential principles. Unless the mother is healthy and carries healthy blood to her conception, the wholeness of health cannot be attained.

Chapter V

CONTINUITY AND HEREDITY

In his Mellon Lecture, in 1922, McCarrison perceived a contrast and sought to explain it. He had come from northwestern India to Pittsburgh, America's city of steel, and he told his hearers in Pittsburgh, as already quoted, that his particular people in north-western India never had the "abdomen over-sensitive to nerve impressions, to fatigue, anxiety, or cold." Indeed, they had no abdominal sensitiveness at all except that of hunger.

Before him was the contrast. "Their buoyant abdominal health," he went on, "has, since my return to the west, provided a remarkable contrast with the dyspeptic and colonic lamentations of our highly-civilized communities." The first were last, and the last first; the forward backward, and the backward forward—what was the reason of this reversal? Another revolution, one would think—some profound revolution of values.

That was not the reason McCarrison gave to his Pittsburgh hearers. To them he gave a practical set of reasons which his audience would appreciate. The first of these was something our particular civilisation had lost. "Infants are reared as nature intended them to be—at the breast. If this source of nourishment fails, they die; and at least they are spared the future of gastro-intestinal miseries which so often have their origin in the first bottle."

Now, the feeding of infants on the breast is clearly as much a part of the whole diet as is the feeding of the fœtus by the mother's blood—with the exception that oxygen is now separated and breathed, and is not a part of the milk as it was of the blood.

Otherwise the breast milk of the Hunza woman is as much derived from Hunza food as is the blood of her womb. Her breast-feeding is only a continuation of the period when she is an intervener between her offspring and the Hunza diet. The breast milk itself is a specially manufactured method of conveying that diet to the child.

The Hunza mother gives the breast for three years. She nourishes the child and protects herself from further pregnancy. To become pregant during lactation is considered unfair to the suckling child, and socially has attached to it a sense of indecency.

Milk, being the purveyor of a diet, is itself a diet. Any one can live on milk. An adult can live on milk only, though he would not have the strength of a man, but that of a child. If he wanted to have the strength of a man on milk he would have to take a very great deal and have the big belly and the other inconvenience of the well-fed baby, but it would be possible.

There is no other thing that is the exact counterpart of milk. The breast takes the nutriment as it is circulating in the mother's blood for her own good in the normal way of things, and separates out a pleasant-looking fluid. This milk is a liquid preparation of foods made by the mother. Except as regards oxygen, it is practically the same as the maternal blood which fed the fœtus in the womb.

This, I think, shows the very vital importance of breast-feeding. It is a continuation. The same process which was going on in the womb is still going on. The radical change at birth was not a change of foods, but a partial change of method. The oxygen which was previously supplied by the maternal blood is now supplied by the child's own lungs. But the character of the foods remains the same. It is a typical continuity, such as is the salvation of anything young and delicate; it is a sheltering of young tissues by repetition and familiarity.

Any change in the nature of the foods, therefore, is risky and alters the line of life. Such a change does not occur in Hunza, says McCarrison. If anything unusual happens, it is the failure of the thing as a whole. It just ends.

A change is risky, and it in itself may well bring life down to a lower physical level from the time it takes place; to the level

of those "dyspeptic and colonic lamentations" which often start
with the first bottle.

How risky is the break in continuity is really astonishingly
shown in figures quoted by the League of Nations Committee on *The Problem of Nutrition* from which we also
quoted in regard to caries of the teeth in the last chapter.

"Complete breast-feeding of infants is of very great
importance," reports the Committee. "Impressive evidence of
this was supplied by a large-scale enquiry from the Infant
Welfare Centre of Chicago, in which 20,061 infants attending
the centre between the years 1924-29 were closely followed
up for the first nine months of each infant life. Of these
48.5 per cent were wholly breast-fed, 43 per cent partially
breast-fed, and 8.5 per cent wholly artificially fed. The
artificial feeding was carried out on a definite plan, and
all the infants—artificially fed and otherwise—were attended
by the officials of the centre. The mortality rates of these
different groups of infants were as follows :

	Number of Infants	Total Deaths	Percentage of Deaths of Infants
Wholly Breast-fed ...	9,749	15	0.15
Partially	8,605	59	0.7
Artificially fed	1,707	144	8.4

"It will be seen that the mortality rate among the artificially
fed infants is fifty-six times greater than amongst the breast
fed. The difference in the death-rate between these classes of
infants was largely due to deaths following respiratory infections, and to a less degree, gastro-intestinal and other infections.
Thus, whereas only four out of 9,749 of the breast-fed infants
died of respiratory infections, eighty-two out of the 1,707
artificially-fed infants died from this cause.

"No clearer evidence could be obtained to enforce the
advantages of breast-feeding as compared with artificial
feeding. Similar impressive evidence on the value of breast-
feeding was afforded by the enquiry of the League of Nations
into the causes of infant mortality in six European countries
and four South American countries, which also demonstrated

the part played by bad feeding in infant mortality. Where this mortality was low the digestive troubles usually caused by bad feeding were rare; where it was high, digestive troubles were very prevalent—they were the outstanding cause of death, and it is by reducing them that mortality can be reduced. Conversely, where breast-feeding was general, the 'nutritional peril' was usually small; where artificial feeding predominated, it was great."

It will be noted in this testimony to continuity, that the conclusion drawn is one of mortality. It is the obvious one when that continuity is so badly shattered that the last extremity of the infant's fight for life is reached. The severity of this measure conveys that survivors fail to attain the physical perfection which can be reached by certain groups of men. And if this is missed and poor physique takes its place, how many social, national, and political troubles may thereby be engendered? Who is to measure them? Who is to deny that in these days they seem to have reached a maximum, which threatens the very disruption of our type of civilization? Who can deny that the failure of breast-feeding is but one symptom amongst a number, and that the divorce of the baby from the breast, the divorce of the mate from the hearth and the divorce of society from stability are not associated as regards their profounder causation?

But, it may be maintained, to one stage we have not yet got. We do not let our children who cannot get breast milk die, and that is the custom of the Hunza. "Sooner our low grade of physique and our liability to many diseases than the abandonment of little innocents," we may say.

The position is not so immediately harsh as it at first appears. It does not mean that if the mother fails the baby dies. There are in the joint families in Asia other women prepared to suckle the child. The grandmother may take the place of the mother. Moreover, good breasts suckle more than one child.

Amongst us there is the infant mortality due to ill-feeding, so strongly commented on by the League of Nations Committee. That is not so with the Hunza. Our intentions may be better, but our results are worse. Result has to be placed beside intention to get a view of what is sound humanity. Had we the high physical quality of the Hunza and the men of Sparta, how should we look upon infantile life—as something destined to high physical efficiency or to be preserved, however feeble, at all costs? The hardness of heart of the Spartans in exposing their new-born infants on the hillside was the necessary corollary of the high standard of their efficiency, which permitted Sparta to be an unwalled city for seven centuries. To grow up a weakling amidst such brethren was to bear a constant stigma. It were better not to be born.

So too amongst the Hunza, the child was a child of their tradition or it was nothing. They had no substitute feeding for it. Continuance, by breast-feeding, was the way to the independence of individual life, and there was no other. There was no general sanctity of human life, whatever it chanced to be; only a sanctity of its quality, its holiness in the old sense of health.

The breast milk of the Hunza women must unquestionably be of excellent quality. The breast milk of the mothers under the observation of the Infant Welfare Centre of Chicago must have been superior to any mixture of cow's milk or any patent food which could be supplied. We now come to a question of vital importance to the whole subject of nutrition.

It is this : Could the breast milk of these women of Chicago be made to give sound physique to their offspring? Or, to put it in terms of modern classification : Could a mother of C3 class, if undiseased herself, be enabled to give uterine- and breast feeding which will ensure an A1 baby? Could the relative degeneracy of modern mothers be wiped out in one generation, or is it handed on by heredity? Is it now ingrained in the race and inevitable?

McCarrison's Coonoor rats were not degenerate rats. They had not inherited any physical defects and weaknesses. They could be made degenerate by being given a faulty Indian or British diet. In the published Cantor Lectures there is a photograph of seven of them hung up by their tails, as if they were in a butcher's shop. They are arranged in degrees of plumpness and size from left to right.

The plumpest was fed on Sikh diet prepared and cooked in the native manner. Next comes the rat fed on foods as cooked and taken by the Pathans, then the Mahratta-fed rat, the Goorkha, the Kanarese, the Bengali, and the Madrassi-fed rats.

Each of these rats represented the average of a group of twenty rats fed on the particular diet for 140 days, corresponding to a period of twelve human years. The rats were of the same age, sex-distribution and body weight, under the same hygiene and in similar cages.

In further photographs of live Sikh-fed rats and live rats fed on the foods of poorer class Europeans, the average representative of the twenty Sikh-fed rats, weighing 188 grains, is a bright alert-looking animal; the representative of the poor European diet, weighing 118 grains, is a poor little creature with tired eyes. One photo of him, however, makes him, at first, look the normal, expected rat, were it not placed alongside of the Sikh-fed rat. Then one can compare details, and one sees, for instance, that the poor European-fed rat has fallen arches to his feet and his neck is weak; there is no firm curve from the forehead to the back. One feels that rat would sooner sit and work at a bench or at a desk than make his muscles glow with hard work upon the field.

One rat is healthy and whole, the other is degenerated, which the dictionary defines as "to fall off from the qualities proper to the race or kind; to become of a lower type, physically or morally; to pass from a good to a worse state."

We know that this degeneracy of the representative poor-European rat is acquired from his food. He started the same as the Sikh-fed rat. It was just bad luck, over which he had no control himself, that he fell off from qualities proper to the race, and that bad luck was poor foods.

More than that McCarrison's rats did not show. They showed acquired degeneracy. They did not show whether this acquired degeneracy could be passed on from parents to offspring through heredity.

The reason why they did not show this is that the experiments were not designed to show it, because the general question as to whether characteristics acquired by progenitors can be handed on to progeny had already been settled, though with shades of dubiety still hovering in some minds.

Professor Weismann, some fifty years ago, stated that acquired characteristics could not be inherited. The first speck of life's first step in life is to divide into two definite parts, one of which is to be the individual and the other the permanent characteristics to be handed on to the offspring. The individual and what he is in life does not alter the characteristics he hands on. He is only a temporary carrier of the seed's characteristics; he is in no way, not even in part, one who can alter their primal character by what he does.

For example, if he is a white-skinned man who, by exposure in the tropics, became a brown-skinned man, he will not from a white wife produce a brown-skinned child. But, if he marries a woman of a brown-skinned race, then, of course, he may produce a brown-skinned child. But this is not due to his own acquired brown skin, but to the racial brown skin of his wife.

Weismann also had his rats or rather mice, and for twenty-two generations he cut off their tails with a carving knife. This had absolutely no effect upon the tails of new-born mice. Before they were cut off, from generation to generation they were the same. A great number of other experiments to test this statement of Weismann have since been made. As the question of heredity is of the utmost importance to that of nutrition, it is fortunate that this question of the inheritance of acquired characteristics has been settled.

The sins of the fathers are *not* visited by heredity upon the children. "It is quite impossible to believe that the lives and habits of the parents have a genetical effect upon their children," writes Mr. Eldon Moore, in his book *Heredity, Mainly Human* (1934). Professor J. A. Thomson in his well-known book on *Heredity* (1926) says the same thing with Scotch caution : "There is little or no scientific warrant for our being other than extremely sceptical as to the inheritance of acquired characteristics."

The answer, then, to these all-important questions is that the effects of faulty feeding are not permanent in the race. They are not stamped into the race ineradicably by heredity.

On the contrary, almost at a stride they could be abolished. Treat one generation rightly in the matter of food and bring and keep the next generation within that same correct feeding, and the change would be effected. This, the right nutrition of man, however, is not the whole of the possibility. There is the further question of the right nutrition of the animals and vegetables he eats, which subject will engage our attention towards the end of this thesis.

Meanwhile, we know that the poor-European or poor-Madrassi-fed rat is made the weakling that he is by the food he gets. His degeneracy is acquired. As to man, one sees the same phenomenon in photographs printed with the Cantor Lectures of the Hunza man, the Sikh man, the Mahratta and the Pathan, on the one hand, and the poor Bengali and Madrassi on the other.

Heredity plays no part in the actual physical condition of any of these men and animals photographed. It is food and food only.

There can be a purgatory of ill-being in this life due to ill-feeding. Nowhere is this more evident than in the miserable pariah dogs of Indian cities. They are scavengers, timid and dispirited, ever hoping to snatch a piece of food without hit or kick.

As youngsters on the way to failure they are often so diseased and ill-looking that even an Englishman, with his good feeling towards dogs, rarely gives one a kind word. If he does so, after the first suspicion the dog wags his tail feebly and sends a shy glance of friendliness, which is the ineffable expression of the strange bond that has so long united dog and man.

If this canine smile of the poor beast wins the heart of the Englishman, what is the result? Well-fed and well-cared for, the dog blossoms into a sleek-coated, healthy dog, with all the good-fellowship of his kind.

This happens although the dog belonged to a class of beings who have for centuries suffered the purgatory of ill-feeding and disease without parallel. Yet, provided there is no serious disease, all this degeneracy that seemed riveted to his class rapidly disperses.

Such is the bearing of heredity upon the effects of foods—it is none. Food is a condition—a primary condition—of environment. A good or bad condition of this environment is mainly dependent upon man himself. It is within his power to make almost miraculous changes.

Chapter VI

OTHER WHOLE-DIET EXPERIMENTS

I HAVE been able to find very few whole-diet nutritional experiments other than those of McCarrison to which I have already referred or which have already been described. They were (1) the experiment in which certain north-western Indian diet was given to 1,189 rats for a period corresponding to forty or fifty years in the life of men; (2) the one in which diets composed of foods "usually those in use by the people of India; sometimes actual Indian dietaries" were tested upon 2,243 rats for the same period of forty to fifty years in the human; (3) the experiment in which seven groups of twenty young rats were given Sikh, Pathan, Mahratta, Goorkha, Kanarese, Bengali and Madrassi diets, prepared and cooked after the manner of the people, for a period corresponding to twelve years in the human; (4) the experiment of two similar groups of rats of twenty each, in which one group was given the north-western Indian diet and the other a diet "such is commonly used by the poorer classes in England" for a period corresponding to about sixteen years in the life of man.

The result of the first experiment was an absence of disease; of the second, many diseases; of the third, an order of merit of the seven racial or communal diets; of the fourth, the grading of the diet of the poorer classes in England with that of the poorer Madrassi.

A striking whole-diet experiment was carried out in Denmark in the last year of the War.

The blockade, following the entry of the U.S.A. into the war, put the Danes in a very serious position. Professor Mikkel Hindhede, Superintendent of the State Institute of Food Research, was made Food Adviser to the Danish Government to deal with it.

The problem that faced him was this: Denmark had a population of 3,500,000 human beings and 5,000,000 domestic animals. She was accustomed to import grains from the United States for both. There was now a shortage of grain foods.

The pigs had provided hams and bacon for the English as well as for Danes. In the crisis the question arose : Would it be wise to get rid of the pigs and let men eat the food which otherwise the pigs would eat? Hindhede decided it would be wise, so some four-fifths of the pigs were killed and about one-sixth of the cattle. Their grain food was given to the Danes, and it was given, not in the exact form in which it was given to the pigs—not as bran mash, for instance—but as wholemeal bread with the extra coarse bran that is not put into ordinary wholemeal bread incorporated.

In addition to this bread, or Kleiebrot, which was made official for the whole country, the Danes ate porridge, green vegetables, potatoes and other root vegetables, milk, butter, and fruit. No grain or potatoes were allowed for the distillation of spirits, so there were no spirits. Half the previous quantity of beer was permitted.

As some pigs were left, the people on the farms got meat; the people in the cities—40 per cent of the population—got very little meat. Only the rich could afford beef.

The food regulations were begun in March 1917 and were made stringent from October 1917 to October 1918.

The result of this enforced national diet was a remarkable lowering of the death-rate. The death-rate, which had been 12.5 in 1913, 1914, now fell to 10.4 per thousand, "which is the lowest mortality figure that has been registered in any European country at any time." (Hindehede).

Hindhede puts this impressive result in another way. Taking the average from 1900 to 1916 as 160, in the October to October year it was 66. Even in men over sixty-five the figure fell to 76.

Hindhede attributes this extraordinary rapid and marked change to two things: (1) less meat, (2) less alcohol. He regards the bran as having largely filled the gap of the scanty or absent meat, bran having a good proportion of vegetable meat or protein. He regards the experiment as a triumph for his previous teaching. "The reader knows," he writes in the

Deutsche Medizinische Wochenschrift of March 1920, "how sharply I have emphasised the advantages of a lacto-vegetarian diet. I am not in principle a vegetarian, but I believe I have shown that a diet containing a large amount of meat and eggs is dangerous to the health."

Now, when the Americans exported wheat and barley from the virgin soil of the prairies, about 1870-1880, and drove European farmers to despair by their low prices, the shrewd Danes quickly changed their agricultural methods. They bred pigs and cattle and poultry, and sent bacon and eggs and butter to England. They also became big eaters of meat and eggs themselves. The war forced them to go back to the foods they used to eat before the invasion of American wheat—foods which their forefathers had eaten for centuries. Especially was this the case with bread.

Hindhede lays much emphasis on the change in bread. Before his fiat the Danes ate fine meal bread and wholemeal bread. He made them eat only wholemeal bread with extra bran. Its proportion he gives as 67 per cent rye, 21 per cent oats, and 12 per cent bran.

Except for the bran, which added vegetable meat for those who were animally meatless or meat short, the bread was the good baked bread which "has been the national bread of Denmark for centuries. For ages it was the only bread procurable in the country and even now it is the common form." (Hindhede).

This was the whole diet of the Danes, which in such a short time had such admirable results : wholemeal bread with added bran, green vegetables, potatoes, other root vegetables, fruit, milk and butter; meat variable, but always less than before and in towns scanty; less alcohol.

There is no doubt that Hindhede is justified in claiming that this proved an excellent diet, producing as it did the record low European death-rate in so short a time. He does not make the inference that it was the commercialism of Americans called forth by western needs that first spoilt this diet about half a century ago and that it was only when the war shut out this American commercialism that it was able to reappear.

If looked at carefully, it will be seen that the foods more closely resemble the Hunza and Sikh foods than those of any modern European diet. The Hunza and Sikh eat wholemeal grains, vegetables, fruit, plenty of milk, butter, and not much meat or alcohol.

Yet to show how one must take a diet as a whole and not pick out certain bits of it for praise or blame, one has only to go to other parts of the Danish Empire to find whole diets producing excellent health, which contradict what the Danish Food Adviser thought he had proved. He certainly proved that what the Danes took under his orders was a good diet, but his inference that quantities of meat are bad for the health compared to a lacto-vegetarian diet is disproved by the next enforced whole-diet experiments to be described, which ironically enough occurred in the Danish possessions, the Faroe Islands, Iceland, and Greenland.

These Danish possessions are three isolated lands from which no western civilized person would expect to glean wisdom. But, as we have already seen in the case of food and health, isolation locks up the most valuable secrets. The peoples of these three lands, living either near or actually within the Arctic Circle, offer in three degrees, from Faroe to Greenland, an increasingly animal, bird, fish diet. It must not be called a meat diet; that is inaccurate, as will be seen. It was largely a diet from the sea and with the great health of the sea, a "soil" outside the realm of terrestial man.

The diet of the Faroe Islanders, when they were more isolated than now, was given in a book published by the Edinburgh Cabinet Library in 1840. It was mainly a whole carcase diet of animal, bird and fish. The islanders ate not merely meat, but everything that could be eaten. There was no such thing as offal. They also made the carcases gamey by hanging for weeks and even months. In addition to their whole carcase food they had barley meal, unleavened barley bread, a few vegetables, such as cabbages, parsnips and carrots. They drank milk, beer, and on festive occasions brandy. But the main food was animal, bird and fish.

The islanders numbered a few thousands, were of the same origin as the Icelanders, and were "in general, remarkably intelligent. They are extremely healthy, and live to a great age, and an old man of ninety-three years lately rowed the governor's boat nearly ten miles." One danger they incurred was an epidemic catarrhal fever, such as we call influenza, which "prevails after the arrival of the ships from Denmark in the spring," after the winter's scarcity. It spread rapidly and was sometimes fatal. Otherwise, "but few diseases are prevalent amongst them."

The inhabitants of Iceland offer a similar and even more interesting picture of carcase diet. McCollum and Simmonds, in *The Newer Knowledge of Nutrition* (1929), summarize the chief facts. "This island was settled in the ninth century by colonists from Ireland and Scandinavia, who took with them cattle, sheep, and horses. Their diet was practically carnivorous in nature for several hundred years. Martin Behaïm (quoted by Burton), writing of Iceland about A.D. 1500, stated : 'In Iceland are found men of eighty years who have never tasted bread. In this country no corn is grown, and in lieu fish is eaten.' Burton, quoting Pierce, states that rickets and caries of the teeth were almost unknown in Iceland in earlier times. . . . The health conditions were good and dental caries was unknown until after 1850. Stefansson exhumed ninety-six skulls from a cemetery dating from the ninth to the thirteenth centuries and presented them to Harvard University. They have been described by Hooton (1918), who found no evidence of caries in any of them. There were but three to four defective teeth in the entire series, and these had suffered mechanical injury. During the last half century caries has steadily increased in Iceland."

Modern Iceland has not the isolation of the period which Burton described. There has been great advance in civilization and population. Fifty per cent of the people now live in towns or trading stations. There are four agricultural schools. Potatoes, turnips, and rhubarb are cultivated. Iceland imports the trade-foods, such as flour, sugar, preserved fruits, and tinned foods. Caries has become common, as have many other ailments.

The north-west coast of Greenland, where the Polar Eskimos live, is within the Arctic Circle. It is the most isolated and the least affected by civilization of these three possessions of Denmark.

Some attempts at gardening have been introduced by the Danes, but previously the only vegetable food the Eskimos got was from the profuse but, in species, limited vegetation of the Arctic summer. Otherwise they lived mainly on sea animals and sea birds. There was no offal. They eat everything that could be eaten. When it was frozen, they often ate it raw.

The thick, heavy skin of the narwhal is particularly favoured. The millions of sea birds which visit their coast supply a winter store of meat and eggs.

As a side issue, I cannot but think that their fondness for the skin of narwhal is not insignificant. Professor Hindhede praises bran, the skin of grain; the Greenlanders, the skin of the narwhal; the Chinese and other peoples also eat the skins of animals and birds. Everything living has a skin of some sort to protect it. It protects it by its extra toughness, but also if microbes and other minute enemies do attack, it is there on the frontier that the battle is waged. In and near the skin are marshalled the protective forces. Any creature that eats the skin of vegetables, fruit, or animal, also eats these protective materials marshalled on the frontier, and may benefit in its own protection thereby. Whether such a pretty hypothesis is true or not, there are suggestions that skins possess a peculiar value. The lion does not rip open the skin. He eats it. He first eats the whole covering of the tender flank, then the soft ribs, then lungs, heart, liver, kidneys and abdominal fat. He comes back later for more skin and the meat. He is a whole carcase feeder with a fondness for the skin. The skin and adjacent part of the potato is the best part, as the Irish know. So also is it the case with the carrot, and, it is said, with young marrows, cucumbers, gherkins, artichokes, radishes, and celery. There is, therefore, a little evidence for the hypothesis.

The Eskimos are also exceptionally healthy. "The fact that the Eskimos of this polar tribe have such excellent physique, hair, and teeth, and such superb health without any trace of scurvy, rickets, or other evidence of malnutrition," write McCollum and Simmonds, "is interesting in the light of their restricted and simple diet."

It is also interesting as a counterweight to Hindhede and other nutritionists who plump for the excellent lacto-vegetarian diet. There are other excellent diets, and the whole-carcase one of the polar Eskimos is one of them.

These are the principal healthy, enforced whole-diet experiments. There are a few others which have occurred in remote islands, such as Tristan da Cunha, the inhabitants of which are said to be very healthy.

There have been, however, many experiments on human beings the reverse of the above, namely, of ill-health due to the abandonment of a previous and the enforcement of a new diet. These have been unintentional and undesired by those who cause their enforcement and by those who suffer it. Iceland, with its modern store goods as just given, is a mild example. I will take but one of their graver ones, because it has been watched and very carefully recorded. It is given in these words by McCollum and Simmonds:

"There is no better illustration of the soundness of the views regarding the types of diet which succeed in inducing good nutrition than the experience of the non-citizen Indian of the United States. All who observed the Indians in their primitive state agree that most of them were exceptional specimens of physical development. With few exceptions, however, during two generations they have deteriorated physically. The reason for this is apparently brought to light by a consideration of the kind of food to which they have restricted themselves since they have lived on reservations.

"There is no group of people with a higher incidence of tuberculosis than the non-citizen Indian. As wards of the Government they have been provided with money and land, but have in general shown little interest in agriculture. They have lived in idleness and have derived their food supplies from the agency stores. In addition to muscle cuts of meat they have, therefore, taken large amounts of milled cereal products, syrup, molasses, sugar and canned foods, such as peas, corn, and tomatoes. In other words, they have come to subsist essentially upon a milled cereal, sugar, tuber, and meat diet. On such a regimen their teeth have rapidly become inferior and are badly decayed. They suffer much from rheumatism and other troubles which result from local infections. Faulty dietary habits are, in great measure, to be incriminated for their susceptibility to tuberculosis.

"Other classes of Indians, who have become successful farmers, have not deteriorated as a result of contact with civilization, except in so far as they have suffered from alcohol and venereal infections. The non-citizen Indian has suffered, not because of contact with civilization, but because he has been forced into dietary habits which are faulty."

These are practically all the whole-diet experiments, diets on which men lived healthily or, in the last case, fell from a state of living healthily.

In the writings of the scientific experts on nutrition, there are very numerous part-diet experiments based on synthetic or specially made-up diets, omitting or cutting down the quantity of one or more of the factors which compose a diet. One scientist will cut down the quantity of protein given and watch the effect of this upon animals; another will cut down the fats and note the resulting sicknesses; another will give vegetable or irradiated vegetable fats in place of customary animal fats; another will give a diet in which vitamin A is defective, B is defective, C is defective, and so on.

The experiments are skilfully devised and carried out with consummate technique. They lead to a mass of knowledge about proteins as things in themselves; fats as things in themselves; vitamins as things in themselves; but whether these can be things in themselves and are not really relative to a host of other conditions in nutrition is as yet scarcely considered. McCarrison's statement in the Cantor Lectures, for example, that "the diet of the Sikhs is only health-promoting so long as it is consumed in its entirety," is foreign to all this fragmentation.

Fragmentation, I take it, arises from the invasion and domination of thought by specialists. A piece of required knowledge is isolated and is studied with great technical skill and intensity by a specialist. This simplification of knowledge by devotion to only a fragment of it is suitable to the intelligence of the average man, and, as there are great numbers of average men, it is easy for present-day civilization to cultivate a number of specialists or simplicists, men to whom thinking is simplified by cutting it down to one problem or set of problems, or one technique or even one particular part of a technical process. It is not only a division of labour, but a division of knowledge which leads to the separation of the intellect from the wider reality of life.

Simplicism, the binding of man to one job or one small department of knowledge, affects every branch of modern life and not only science. If one breaks away from one's special box to seek the wide world of knowledge, and thinks to find a way under the tutorage of experts, one soon finds oneself in a Sudanese dust-storm. So finely fragmented is the knowledge, one loses sight of the real world.

I am, however, here only concerned with this fragmentation in the matter of research upon nutrition, and in the argument that diet is a whole thing, already proven in the living world, wherever there are animals and plants, vigorous and without disease.

I shall deal with fragmentation in the next chapter.

Chapter VII

FRAGMENTATION

THE factors of a diet upon which it is now believed life depends will perhaps one day be as many as the notes of a piano. At present there may be said to be thirty.

There are, firstly, the proteins or meaty substances of the food. They have been found to consist of chemical substances called amino-acids. There are eighteen amino-acids known to chemistry. Some of them are necessary to life. Lysin and cystine are necessary; tryptophane is almost certainly so; arginine and histidine, one or the other, but not necessarily both, are so. That gives four factors necessary to life.

Then there are fats and certain lipins they contain. They occur in all foods except sugar and some fruits. To what degree they are essential to life it has not been finally determined, so one factor for fats is sufficient.

The same may be said of starches and sugars, or carbohydrates, to give them their group name. Carbohydrates are the immediate fuel of energy, and fats the stored fuel. Energy is an essential quality of life. Carbohydrates can, then, count as one factor.

These food substances are composed of chemical elements. Of the elements known to exist in the body, some, possibly all, are necessary to life. They are carbon, hydrogen, nitrogen, oxygen, potassium, sodium, iron, copper, manganese, zinc, magnesium, lithium, phosphorus, sulphur, chlorine, iodine, barium, silicon. They add eighteen factors and raise the total number to twenty-four.

These elements are not only combined to form proteins, fats, carbohydrates, but they also form the mineral salts of the body, the chlorides, phosphates, carbonates, sulphates and so on, of sodium, potassium, calcium, iron, and so on. We will not add anything for the mineral salts, but allow them to be grouped under the eighteen elements.

Another set of substances necessary to life are the vitamins. Vitamins A, B1, B2, C, D are necessary to life. There are other vitamins, buds, as it were, from B called B3, B4, B5, B6, also E and somewhat nebulous vitamins up to K. It is safe to say that five vitamins are essential to life.

Lastly, there is water, which brings the total number of dietary factors necessary to life to thirty.

These necessities have been found out by giving animals diets in which one of the factors was missing. If the animals did not die, the factor was not necessary to their lives. It might be necessary to their health; they might live feebly without it. They might get a particular disease without it. This led to a further mass of research on these particular factors of disease. Then there have been experiments to find out which of two or more factors of like type was the best. Thus a great deal has been learnt about a factor or group of factors as separate things.

Let us take, for example, the proteins or meaty foods. The first protein to be isolated and separated as a thing or substance in itself was gelatin. Gelatin, therefore, became the object of a great deal of nutritional research.

Firstly dogs were tested out on gelatin, as the only protein of an otherwise complete diet, by Voit, over fifty years ago. But gelatin failed to fill the full protein needs, and the dogs got thinner day by day. There was something lacking in gelatin as a full necessary protein food.

Proteins build up and replace the tissues of the body and supply the necessary element, nitrogen. Gelatin failed to do this on its own. It could do it in part, but there was a gap in its completeness.

When it was found that proteins were made up of amino-acids, this gap proved very useful to the research workers. By putting a particular amino-acid into the gap its efficiency could be tested.

Kessels, in 1905, tried the first of these experiments. Dogs, Voit found, starve if given gelatin as their only source of nitrogen. Kessels gave dogs gelatin plus such amino-acids as tyrosine, cystine, and tryptophane. The dogs lived. He then fed himself in the same way, and found he could carry on quite well. So the gap in gelatin was successfully filled.

By experiments like this the amino-acids were eventually ranged in order of value. Some failed to fill the gap, and the weight of the dogs continued to be lost. Some succeeded, and prevented the loss. With growing animals, some succeeded better than others in filling the gap, as shown by the normal increase of weight. In this way an order of merit of the amino-acids was created.

From the separate amino-acids it was easy to pass to the separate proteins. There are so many of them in the vegetable and animal worlds and they vary so much according to how many amino-acids they contain and how they are arranged that work on this subject could be endless. Berg, for example, in 1903, calculated that the number of possible proteins, based on the amino-acids, was 6,708,373,705,728,100. So research workers were driven to test out the best known ones.

There is a chart in McCollum and Simmonds' book which is quite exciting in its effect. It is like the start of a horse race. Nice thick black lines, indicating the weights of experimented rats, leap forwards from the base line into the air together. The rat that leaped highest was not quite a fair starter, being given two proteins, those of rye and flax-seed meal, whereas the remaining rats were only given one protein-containing food in a made-up diet. The next starter, not much behind the rye and flax-seed candidate in his leap was milkfed. Then came wheat, rye, maize, flax-seed alone, barley, oats, and Kaffir corn-fed rats.

By experiments of this kind the proteins can be arranged in order of worth; in the same way as McCarrison arranged the *whole* diets as prepared and eaten by the Sikhs, Pathans, Mahrattas, Goorkhas, Kanarese, Bengalis and Madrassis. By the former experiments you find out which are the best, or probably best, proteins for a diet which you are putting together under expert advice; or which, as an expert, you will advise for others. It settles for you one factor of diet, the proteins.

There are the many other known factors to be considered, as well as the need to keep a watch on new discoveries. The vitamins, for example, first appeared some forty years ago, when Eijkman of Batavia published the results of his investigations on the paralysis of fowls fed on polished rice. They have led to a great increase of knowledge. They are by no means the end. There are "countless substances in food," Sir Gowland Hopkins wrote in 1906. There must needs be other important unknown factors yet to be discovered.

Meanwhile, experts can tell us what happens to animals and humans who do not get sufficient vitamin A. The most dramatic is dry eyes, leading to blindness, but if fresh vitamin is quickly given there is a miraculous recovery. Or there are the troubles which do not clear up miraculously, but yet are due in part to defective vitamin A. Such are colds, bronchitis, pneumonia, and weakness of the bowels. So one has to keep a watch on one's supply of vitamin A.

Vitamin B effects miracles no less wonderful. There is nothing more dramatic in nutritional research than a common experiment which was often carried out in a laboratory where I worked. A pigeon deprived of the needed vitamin B by being kept on polished rice is lying on the floor of its cage, unable to rise. It may be contorted in a remarkable manner, bent right backwards, like one of the living croquet hoops in *Alice in Wonderland,* or forwards as if doubled up between two invisible hands. It may suddenly be released from these spasms only to be thrown into violent convulsions. It is near to death and will in fact soon die if left.

But if one takes a glass tube, puts into it the pulp of some sprouting pulse or grain, prizes open the pigeon's beak, and blows the pulp down its throat, the miracle happens. In a very short time the pigeon is its usual self, on its perch and preening its ruffled feathers.

No experiment can persuade the onlooker more convincingly of the power of a vitamin than can this one. That is because it is dramatic. But there are many forms of ill-health due to poor supply of B which are not at all obvious.

Then there is vitamin C. Animals and men deprived of

vitamin C get into the most deplorable condition with foul, bleeding mouths, bleeding elsewhere and eventual death—the terrible disease of scurvy. This is an easy disease to prevent. It is very rare to see it now, but minor degrees of the scurvy condition, with its weakness, headaches, poor appetites, affected gums—they are common. Moreover, vitamin C is not like the other vitamins. They are, like common salt and other substances, not notably altered by ordinary heat or storage. But vitamin C is. It is volatile and unstable in character. It is, therefore, apt to be deficient in a diet which varies according to the supply of things in season, and most urban diets are like this.

So we could continue with further vitamins, and if desired, make another procession through the mineral salts, giving details of the astonishing amount of experiments there have been and information gathered on each several part of our food.

We learn what are the best proteins, what the best fats, the best carbohydrates, the best sources of calcium, phosphorus, iron and other minerals, of vitamin A, vitamin B, and so on, until we are or should be able to select our diet, not by taste, as we do in a restaurant, but by knowledge. We shall in this way do our best to fulfil the wish expressed by McCollum and Simmonds, namely, "the discovery of the means of making nice adjustments in a qualitative way among all the factors best adapted to promote optimum development."

The method of proceeding to the optimum development by fragmentation, that is, breaking up of food into its several elements and by experiment discovering a great deal about each fragment and then putting them together in a better way, is a method that could only spring out of certain conditions. It could only spring from disease, not health. If our diet gave us health we should not question it. But it does not do so. On the contrary, there has been so much disease in the last one or two centuries that we began to question many things as possible causes of the ill-health. Amongst them we questioned our diet. In doing so our scientists have taken it to pieces as a machine is taken to pieces, and carefully

examined each piece as regards its suitability. They have fragmented it, and now the time of synthesis approaches, the
putting it together again. Here, however, they are far much
less certain than they were in fragmentation, which continues
to possess them, with the consequence that each fragment gets
boosted as occasion arises; we are told to eat more potatoes,
eat more fruit, eat more home-grown meat, drink more milk,
drink more beer, take more salt or less salt, be careful to
take milk for vitamin A, green vegetables for vitamin B,
fresh fruit for vitamin C—all well-studied fragments, but fragments nevertheless.

All this knowledge would be quite useless to the Hunza
people. They have, for long, found a diet that is "adapted
to promote optimum development." They have formed it out
of foods not widely different from European foods, for, as
McCarrison says in the Cantor Lectures : "Things nutritional
are not, in essence, so different in India and in England."

The chief difference is that they have a settled traditional
diet into which they are born and a settled traditional way
of growing it and caring for it. They have a whole system,
a diet as a whole thing, whole not only in itself, but in its
history, its culture, its storage, and its preparation.

And with their whole diet they preserve the wholeness of
their health. This also we have failed to do. Our health or
wholeness has fragmented no less than our diet. A swarm of
specialists have with the invention of science settled on the
fragments to study them. A great deal is found out about
each several disease; there is a huge, unmanageable accumula-
tion of knowledge, and this and that disease is checked or overcome. But our wholeness has not been restored to us. On the
contrary, it is fragmented into a great number of diseases and
still more ailments. We have lost wholeness, and we have got
in its place its fragmentation with a multiplexity of methods,
officially blessed and otherwise, dealing with the fragments in
their severalty.

Chapter VIII

THE CAUSATION OF DISEASE

SIR EDWARD E. MELLANBY, in his book *Nutrition and Disease,* quotes experiments he undertook with Dr. A. H. Green designed to prove that ill-fed rats were very liable to infections.

The diet which he gave them was a laboratory synthetic diet so prepared as to show what happens when one kind of food is defective. In this case the defective fragment was vitamin A.

Although the diet was not a whole diet, such as certain groups of men eat, nevertheless the results are of great interest in showing how this particular faulty diet can be the primary cause of a large group of diseases. Mellanby states that Green and he found areas of infections in almost all the ninety-two young rats brought up on this diet.

These areas of infection due to the same cause were very varied in character and situation. One rat would have something wrong with its ear, another with its stomach, another with its bladder, and so on. So different were the infective conditions found that one is not surprised that a practical man would roughly give each a separate cause. Actually 44 per cent of the 92 rats had something wrong with their urinary organs; 24 per cent with their ears and noses; 38 per cent with their eyes; 21 per cent with their stomachs and intestines; and 9 per cent with their lungs.

These abscesses and infections only occurred in the rats if they were given defective vitamin A; if given proper food, they did not occur. Mellanby's words are: "If a source of vitamin A, such as butter, cod liver oil or egg yolk formed a part of the diet, infective lesions were never seen in the rats, the addition of these substances to the deficient diets, unless the animals were too severely infected, generally resulted in rapid improvement and ultimate cure."

These experiments upon an important fragment of diet exhibit correspondingly a part of the results of McCarrison's Coonoor rats when fed on the poorer Bengali and Madrassi diets. The rats of Coonoor got all these infections and a good deal more, as we have seen. But Mellanby's results show, in the same way as McCarrison's more extensive experiments, that in the infections of rats fed with deficient vitamin A the primary cause of the infections is shifted from the microbes to food. As a primary cause of these diseases the position of the microbes were undermined. Something deeper in causation was found.

The diseases of 2,243 group of Coonoor rats, and some other animals used at Coonoor, must here be repeated. They got diseases of the respiratory system, adenoids, pneumonia, bronchitis, pleurisy, pyothorax and infections of the nose; infections of the ear; infections of the eye; dilated stomach, growths, ulcer and cancer of the stomach, inflammation of the small and large gut; constipation and diarrhœa; diseases of the urinary passage, such as Bright's disease, stone, abscesses, inflammation of the bladder; inflammation of the womb and ovaries, death of the fœtus, premature birth, hæmorrhage; diseases of the testicles; inflammation of the skin, loss of hair, ulcers, abscesses, gangrene of the feet and tail; anæmias of the blood; enlarged lymphatic glands, cystic and suppurating glands; goitre and diseases of the special glands; wasting, enlargement of and inflammation of the muscle, and inflammation of the outer lining of the heart; inflammation and degeneration of the nervous tissues; diseased teeth and bones; dropsy; scurvy; feeble growth, feeble appetite, weakness, lassitude, and ill-temper.

"All these conditions," said McCarrison, in the Cantor Lectures, "these states of ill-health, had a common causation; faulty nutrition with or without infection."

One wonders whether, with the exception of plague, these small animals could get any more diseases than those of this formidable list. I do not know if anyone has discovered how many diseases rats can get, but they cannot be expected to get all the diseases of the more complicated man. Nevertheless, one cannot assert that poor food so breaches the barrier to disease of rats that every disease which they get can swarm into the stronghold of their health, as invaders swarmed into a mediæval city when the walls had been breached, to destroy it in a number of ways and scattered localities. But one can say that a great number of the rat's diseases do so, or in other words that poor food in rats is the primary cause of a great portion of disease in them.

In minimising this astounding, but in a sense obvious, conclusion, one could say that what is true for rats is not necessarily true for man. That, as a fact, is what Sir John Orr in *Food, Health and Disease* (1936) does say about the rats of Coonoor: "Such experiments with rats, of course, do not carry the same weight as observations of human beings."

This criticism is particularly interesting because it follows, not only a brief précis of McCarrison's work, but also one of a valuable, similar and later experiment of Orr's upon rats fed upon "the average diet eaten by a working-class community in Scotland (with its) daily variation, thus mimicking the food habits of human beings." There was, however, a small addition to the quantities of milk, as the rats could not be bred without the larger allowance (*Journal of Hygiene,* Vol. 35). The results were in the main similar to those of McCarrison.

Now, the noticeable thing about this criticism is that Orr fragments the experiments of both McCarrison and himself. It separates the experiments upon rats from the observations of human beings.

In actual fact McCarrison's experiments were preceded by and due to observations upon human beings. The men were observed first and then the rats. Orr's experiments were due to the example of McCarrison and observations of the unsatisfactory state of the Scotch working-class. Ill-health was transferred to rats by men's faulty food. Without the observations of men the experiments would never have been undertaken.

The criticism shows the hold fragmentation has upon the mental habits of scientists. Orr no sooner reaches McCarrison's truth by his own experiment than he separates himself from it owing to this habit.

A further comment might be made, namely, that the food would never have had such a full effect if the healthy rats had not been cleanly and airily housed and enjoyed sheltered lives, even though these conditions were also those of the sickly rats.

Air, or rather oxygen, it can rightly be maintained, is a part of the food. When the human being is in the womb, oxygen is not separated in any way from the other elements of food, but is brought with them by the mother's blood. It remains a food after birth, but it has peculiar importance in assisting at so many vital processes of movement and energy that it has constantly to be sprayed into the blood by the special apparatus of the lungs.

Hence the airy cages of the rats of Coonoor were a healthy asset, but that is all. They did not save the sickly rats. Further, a number of animals do not live in the fresh air. They go out into it for their food, but they live in burrows and holes. The rats do. So in effect do the Hunza in two winter months. But they also go out into the best of air.

As to sanitary hygiene, that of the Hunza could not compare with that of the rats of Coonoor.

The inescapable conclusion is that in a very large number of diseases faulty food is the primary cause. The suspicion is that faulty food is the primary cause of such an overwhelming mass of disease that it may prove to be simply *the primary cause of disease*.

Up to the present day, it seems, the medical profession and the public have had to be satisfied with a fragmentation of causation, that is to say, a very great number of secondary causes and often enough no real causes at all, but causes as fictitious as they are popular.

For the purposes of illustrating and emphasising the really immeasurable importance of this contrast, if correct, let us take some few of these illnesses and put their causes as given in medical text-books and as shown by the rats of Coonoor in parallel columns.

Let us first take that dangerous disease, pneumonia. Pneumonia is due to a microbe, the pneumococcus, which is found in masses in the lung in true lobar pneumonia. The pneumococcus, says the text-book, is a resident of the human mouth. It is found in 80 to 90 per cent of normal, healthy individuals. Something more, then, than the mere presence of the pneumococcus must be the cause of pneumonia; something that makes this domesticated microbe suddenly become dangerous. In other words, the pneumococcus cannot be called the primal cause of pneumonia. Something has to precede it—some weakness of the barrier.

The weakness of old age is given first of the orthodox causes in the text-book. That beloved physician the late Sir William Osler, whose famous text-book is now under the competent care of Dr. Thomas McCrae, called pneumonia rather charmingly "the friend of the aged"—saving them "the cold gradations of decay."

Pneumonia is more common in cities than in the country and in males than in females. Any weakening habit, such as that of over-drinking, becomes a cause, and also makes the microbes more lethal. Yet robust men may be attacked. Cold is a cause if it weakens, but not if a man finds it a tonic and reacts to it. A previous attack makes a second attack more probable. Another illness, such as chronic kidney or heart disease or one of the acute infectious fevers, gives opportunity to the pneumococcus. So also pneumonia may follow a blow on the chest.

Now let us place these causes from text-books in juxtaposition with that of the "small universe" of Coonoor.

CAUSES OF PNEUMONIA

TEXT BOOKS	COONOOR
Weakness of old age.	Faulty food.
Debilitating habits.	
Exhaustion.	
Chill.	
Previous attack.	
Some other illness, chronic or acute.	
A blow on the chest.	
Pneumococcus microbe.	

The text-books' causes are all more or less of one kind. They may be called secondary weaknesses.

Old age, for instance, is a secondary weakness. Old age

was not permitted to the rats of Coonoor. They were allowed to live by the terms of the experiments to the comparative age of forty or fifty human years, but not to seventy or ninety. But the Hunza confront old age, not with illnesses, but with a vigour that is more like that of youth. We have recorded Skrine's account of their Mir playing polo with skill and activity when nearly seventy, and Schomberg writes of him, when about seventy-five, as being consoled for the death of his Benjamin through a gun accident by other "olive branches" who had happily appeared.

Of debilitating habits, the text-books put alcoholism in the first place. The Hunza, about 1880, when Biddulph wrote his *Tribes of the Hindoo Koosh*, were, he said, "great wine drinkers," and an affront to more orthodox Moslem neighbours, who did not drink at all, and may well have exaggerated the Hunza habit. But at no time were they drunkards. That would be impossible in their precipitous country. McCarrison speaks of them as very moderate in their drinking.

Exhaustion was and is also unknown in Hunza in the meaning it has in the text-books. For example, Schomberg's attendant's horse was stolen. The owner "went after it and kept up the pursuit in drenching rain over mountains for nearly two days with bare feet." There is no hesitation in these sort of acts. Their physique is ready, their apprehension of exhaustion practically nil.

Chills, too, cannot play a part in Hunza life as extra-ordinary and debilitating effects. They endure the winter and its gales at 8,000 feet. Schomberg tells of a Hunza who used to make a hole in the ice on either side of a broad pond. He dived in at one hole, swam under the ice, and came out at the other for enjoyment.

Previous attacks of diseases, the existence of chronic disease of the heart or kidney, or acute infectious diseases, cannot play much part as causes of other illnesses, such as pneumonia, where disease generally is rare. A blow on the chest may also be put aside.

Summing up the text-books' causes, one may call them a number of added weaknesses to an inferior barrier against disease. The barrier gives way readily at this or that point. In other words, the barrier has degenerated.

By his skilled science man is actually able to get a partial picture of what this barrier is. It is in fact an actual barrier. It can be seen through the microscope. It can be seen if it looks healthy or degenerate. It can be photographed, and the photograph of a healthy barrier has clear outlines and demarcations and that of a degenerate barrier is blurry. This barrier is the fine skin which lines the tubes and cells of the nose, windpipe and bronchial tubes, of the mouth, throat, stomach and small and large gut. This fine interior skin is much the same as the outer skin of the body, only it is thinner and softer. But both have an outer layer of cells called epithelium, and it is the epithelium that can be particularly well seen under the microscope. It is the epithelium that forms the visible barrier and which shuts out microbes and other intruders. It does not by any means form the whole barrier, but it constitutes a part of it, which can be seen as clear and definite or blurred and indefinite, according to whether it is itself well or ill fed. The contrast picture gives anyone with even a little knowledge of the microscope a good idea of what can be termed the barrier or, more accurately, the first line of defence. It is not fiction.

So we can understand how it is that faulty food can stand alone under the heading Coonoor against the juxtaposed text-books' list of the causes of pneumonia. It can be placed there as primary, and thereby able to make all the causes in the text-books possible; it can activate them. Without it they would be inert.

Now let us look at the common infection of the middle ear. Mellanby found this infection in a fifth of his faultily-fed rats. It was common among the ill-fed rats of Coonoor, but absent in the well-fed. On the other hand, a well-known text-book, such as Politzer's *Diseases of the Ear*, does not mention faulty food as a cause, any more than faulty food was mentioned under pneumonia. That the whole basis of modern life may be wrong and that that is why such large text-books have to be written has not as yet appeared in the text-books themselves.

Putting the causes of acute infection of the middle ear into juxtaposed columns, we have :—

TEXT BOOKS	COONOOR
External atmospheric conditions	Faulty food
Colds in the head.	
Infectious diseases, such as measles, pneumonia and influenza.	
Sea baths.	
Nasal douches.	

There must, therefore, in faultily fed people be a fear of cold night air, colds in the head; other people coughing and sneezing; schools where children mingle with children; bathing in the sea, and keeping off the "flu" by snuffing lotions or using nasal douches, as recommended by advertisers. Any of these things may lead to passing of the barrier and the defences of the tissues of the ear.

The eyes are even more commonly affected by faulty food than the ears. The sickly rats of Coonoor got inflammations of the eyes, ulcers, and a particular "dry" eye leading to blindness. All of these the well-fed rats escaped.

The text-books all accept defective food as a cause of "dry" eye or xerophthalmia, and recommend cod liver oil and butter, which will cure it if not too far advanced. With this exception there is no direct reference to faulty food as a cause of diseases of the eye. There is only the general statement that these diseases are more common among the poor and debilitated.

A medico-surgical disease which is of particular interest is peptic ulcer, or ulcer of the stomach or duodenum. It is of particular interest because of its proven direct relation to faulty food. It happens to be very common amongst the poorer classes of Southern Travancore—so common that both Lt.-Col. Bradfield, I.M.S., and Dr. Somervell asked McCarrison to put rats on the foods as prepared and eaten by these people. He

put a batch of rats on the foods as prepared and cooked by
the poorer folk of Southern Travancore for 675 days, and at
the end of that time peptic ulcer was found in over a quarter
of them.

This striking result has not yet appeared in the text-books.
As is the way of new knowledge, it passes into currency by a
process of slow percolation. Until the time comes when it
reaches the text-books the causes of peptic ulcer, placed in
juxtaposition, appear as follows:

CAUSES OF PEPTIC ULCER

Text Books	Coonoor
Occupation: anæmic and dys-peptic servant girls, shoe-makers, surgeons.	Primarily faulty food. Specifically such food as that of the poorer classes of Southern Travancore.
Injury.	
Associated diseases such as anæmia, heart d i s e a s e, diseases of liver, appendix, gall bladder, teeth, tonsils.	
Nervous strain.	
Disturbances of the circulation.	
Large superficial burns.	
Certain families are said to be more liable.	
Increased acidity of the stomach.	
Several of the above in combination.	

The last disease I propose to take in these few illustrations
is tuberculosis. As regards this dreaded disease, McCarrison,
in the Cantor Lectures, turned from his own work to one of
the most remarkable of human experiments, that of the Papworth Settlement, so intimately associated with the name of
Sir Pendrill Varrier-Jones.

Papworth is a settlement for sufferers from tuberculosis,
mostly in the form of consumption of the lungs. The patients
are, of course, ill when they come to the settlement, but under
a care, really quite like that given to the rats of Coonoor,
namely, adequate food supply, good housing and ventilation

and freedom from anxiety in the form of loss of employment, there are remarkable and sustained recoveries.

All patients at Papworth have sputum pots and pocket flasks into which they must spit. The infected sputum is at once made innocuous. Moreover, public opinion in the village enforces their use by attaching shame, not to the users, but to those who dare to be forgetful.

In Papworth there are many married couples. The children of these couples live in the settlement. They are in frequent contact with tuberculosis and are protected from the disease by the general use of the spitting pots and flasks and by good food, or, in Varrier-Jones's own words: "the child's resistance to disease is maintained by (a) adequate nutrition, and (b) the absence of mass dose of infection."

Now comes the outstanding fact. The Papworth village has been in existence twenty years, yet not one of the children of these married couples has developed any form of tuberculosis. "Our experience proves," writes Sir Pendrill in his report for 1936, "that no tuberculosis disease need be transmitted so long as village settlement conditions of housing and employment are properly utilised. Any question of 'heredity' is now generally discredited."

In face of this testimony to the power of resistance to tuberculosis given by good food and housing, and with spitting pots to avoid mass infection, the text-books put forward 'predisposition' as a widely-accepted medical tenet.

The argument for predisposition or diathesis runs as follows. Nearly all dwellers in cities can be shown by careful tests to have had minor attacks of tuberculosis. The reason why some persons get the disease and perhaps succumb, whereas the majority are not aware that they have ever been attacked, is that some people have a predisposition to the disease or a diathesis. They are born, so to speak, with an unhappy title to it, or, as the tenet is expressed by Professor Karl Pearson: "the diathesis of pulmonary tuberculosis is certainly inherited, and the intensity of the inheritance is sensibly the same as that of any normal physical character yet investigated in man. Infection probably plays a necessary part, but in the artisan classes of the urban population of England it is doubtful if their members can escape the risks of infection, except by the absence of diathesis—*i.e.* the inheritance of what amounts to a counter-disposition."

Against Papworth's nutrition and avoidance of mass infection is set the medical dogma or tenet of diathesis, or inherited predisposition.

This terrible Calvinistic doctrine, by which certain people, and particularly artisans of the cities, are born predestined to get tuberculosis has therefore been challenged by the good food, security, and the avoidance of mass infection at Papworth.

The Papworth results suggest the following juxtaposition:

CAUSES OF TUBERCULOSIS

TEXT BOOKS	PAPWORTH
Infection with tubercle bacilli.	Inadequate nutrition.
Inherited predisposition.	Mass doses of infection.
Living in dark, close alleys and tenement houses, excess of alcohol and other weakening habits.	
Confinement in prisons, work-houses and workshops.	
Catarrh of respiratory passages.	
Diabetes, kidney disease and other chronic affections which lower resistance.	

If the list of the text-book is carefully examined, we see how the causes there given are all, except that of diathesis, to be found contained in the two Papworth causes. Infection with the tubercle bacilli in the one column is duplicated by the mass infection of the other. Frequent inhalation of quantities of the microbes gives greater opportunities to them to breach the barriers. All the rest are the fragmentation of "inadequate nutrition."

Living in dark, close alleys and tenements means also faulty food. The impure air of slums means one food, namely, oxygen, being defective, but it means also that people who breathe it have not the money for foods that cannot, like oxygen, be got for nothing. Alcohol in excess destroys the appetite. So do the poisons of such diseases as diabetes and kidney disease. So does confinement in prisons, workhouses and workshops. None of the people debilitated by such places or such diseases eat heartily of good food. As to catarrh of the respiratory passages, that in itself was produced by McCarrison and also by Mellanby by faulty food. The barrier breaks down before the catarrhal microbes. A mass attack of tubercle bacilli may do the rest.

If, then, one can put aside the predestination theory of tuberculosis, there lies one thing behind all the other causes given, and that is faulty food and, moreover, as we shall see, faulty food may account for the apparent predestination.

That is sufficient discussion of particular diseases to show the contrast of causes. To discuss more of them would be to enter the maelstrom where diseases are regarded as separate entities, with their individual causes, each one the source of an effervescence of research.

These Papworth children were quoted because they proved heretics to the medical tenet of predestination in tuberculosis and by implication in more than tuberculosis. They might also have been quoted as examples of the making of sound general health, for they have good barriers to disease generally, as the annual reports testify. But if their good health and freedom from tuberculosis breaks or helps to break the tenet of predestination, that in itself will be a specific triumph of almost immeasurable importance.

Fortunately there is another triumph in establishing the general cause of many diseases and ill-healths in poor English children. With just as unpromising human material as that of the Papworth children, the late Miss Margaret MacMillan gained this success, which is described in her book *The Nursery School* (1930).

The MacMillan Nursery School is in Deptford, in the south-east district of London. The school consists of two hundred and sixty children of the Deptford slums, adopted when two years old and kept until fifteen. These children are cared for in a number of ways which reflect the imaginative sympathy of the mind of the directress and the practical embodiments of which would take too long to describe. Among the methods of care is, of course, well-considered food.

Next door to the school is "our own" Deptford Clinic for sick children. School and clinic under the one authority present themselves as human replicas of the rats of Coonoor.

Here is Miss MacMillan's description of the food of the school. "Out all day in moving air, children are always hungry at meal-times, but no food is given between meals. In summer they have fruit from the old mulberry-tree, and we give small spoonfuls of orange juice. Fruit and fresh vegetables are needed by everyone, but especially by growing children, and most of all by children of the poorest classes in cities. Their bones are literally starved of mineral salts. They suffer from starvation in the way of nitrogenous food and of all that nature supplies in green food and fruits. Bread, bread, and always bread in surfeit is their portion. Our fresh vegetables, meal, and milk work wonders."

The test of a diet is the wholeness of those who eat it. This is the description of the children of seven, after four years spent in the school: "They are all straight, well-grown children, and the average is a well-made child, with clean skin, alert, sociable, eager for life and new experience. . . . The abyss between him and the child of yesterday yawns deepest, perhaps when we compare the *state* rather than the achievements of the nurtured child with that of the other. The nurtured seven year old is a stranger to clinics; he knows very little about doctors. He sees the dentist, but has hardly ever, or perhaps never, needed any dental treatment."

To "our clinic" come the sick children of Deptford. They are just ordinary poor children who go to other schools and have other homes than hers. They present the picture of the sickly rats of Coonoor; Miss MacMillan draws the contrast, though not in juxtaposed columns.

"There, ranged on seats by the walls, sit scores of sufferers. Blepharitis, impetigo, conjunctivitis, skin diseases of many kinds—these are not seen in our school. They are seen in the clinic—thousands of cases all preventable." There follow further illnesses seen in the clinic—adenoids, tonsils, colds, coughs, bronchitis, enlarged glands, gastric and intestinal troubles—in short, the list which afflicted the sickly rats of Coonoor.

Now both Sir Pendrill Varrier-Jones and Miss MacMillan have been exceptionally imaginative in seeing that *all* the conditions of life in those under their care were made wholesome, things of the mind as well as those of the body, and it is to this wholeness that they attribute the health of their wards. They do not select food as the primary cause of the health. They regard the whole as resulting in health.

This is so reasonable that I think no one reading their results would care to diminish any one guard of healthy life which they have erected, such as modern housing and hygiene.

Yet, apart from proofs and arguments already put forward to maintain the vital primary claim of food, there is one very exquisite human experiment made by Dr. G. C. M. M'Gonigle, Medical Officer of Health of Stockton-on-Tees, which strengthens this claim in a manner that may be called one of accidental finality.

Stockton-on-Tees is an ancient market town which has grown rapidly in the last three quarters of a century and now has a population of 67,722 (1931). Of this population in that year 40 per cent of the males between fourteen and sixty-five were unemployed.

Stockton has slums, and the Town Council recently carried out a vigorous policy of better housing. It was this that gave M'Gonigle an opportunity to exercise his excellent powers of scientific observation.

A survey of housing needs was taken in 1919, and the largest section of the town scheduled as an unhealthy area was dubbed "Number 1 area." It was decided to demolish a part of Number 1 and transfer its inhabitants to a new up-to-date municipal estate, agreeably named Mount Pleasant. In 1927, 152 families, comprising 710 individuals, were transferred to Mount Pleasant, leaving behind in Number 1 area 289 families with a total of 1,298 individuals.

Here, then, were contrasting conditions of new and old, of good housing and slum. Naturally everyone thought the transfer to Mount Pleasant would be a betterment. But M'Gonigle watched.

Even he, however, watched at first according to the routine of his official position. It was only when he found that something odd was happening and the expected success was not coming off, that he concentrated a keen and skilled observation upon the anomaly.

His attention was drawn to it by the fact that the health of the inhabitants of Mount Pleasant, instead of improving or at least remaining stationary, began to deteriorate, whereas that of those families and people left behind in the slums did not.

M'Gonigle then began to test out what was happening statistically. The standardized death-rate of the first five years following upon the transfer was 33 per 1,000; that of the unchanged slum 22 per thousand. The rate for the Mount Pleasant estate of "33.55 per thousand, appears to be extraordinary, in view of the fact that it represents an increase of 46 per cent over the mean standardised rates for the same individuals in the previous quinquennium," is M'Gonigle's comment. The increase was not due to any peculiarity of infant mortality, epidemic, or other recognized cause. It was just there steadily throughout, and it represented an increase in the various groups, from 0 to 10, between 10 and 65, and over 65. There was even an increase of one-third in still birth. It was a characteristic of the whole people of Mount Pleasant. It was "a real increase and beyond the probable extent of fortuitous variation."

What was it due to? The better housing? It seems absurd that something better should prove something worse. Yet, in spite of the best intentions, this happens if primary things are forgotten. Man lives primarily by food, not by housing, and the food of the Mount Pleasant people was what had deteriorated.

When living in the slums these people paid rents which averaged 4/8 a week per family. In 1928, on the Mount estate, the rent was 9/- a week, and by 1932 it had risen to 9/3½ per week, or double the original rent.

Consequently there was less money to spend on food.

M'Gonigle worked out the average amount spent on food per individual for Mount Pleasant and for slum by carefully prepared and corrected statistics. It is obvious, in view of the different rents paid, that Mt. Pleasant was worse off. Particularly was this shown in the case of unemployed of both areas. The food per "man" per week in Mount Pleasant cost 34.7 pence, that in the unchanged slum, 45.6 pence.

M'Gonigle was, therefore, forced to the conclusion that the deterioration of food led to the deterioration of health. "Such environmental factors as housing, drainage, overcrowding or insanitary conditions" could obviously be excluded. These secondary factors were not worse at Mount Pleasant. They were a great deal better. That was the good fortune of this illuminating experiment. The secondary things, namely, housing and sanitation, were made better first, and in making them better money was withdrawn from the individual's primary need—food.

The experiment emerges as an indictment of putting the building of new houses and of organizing physical drill on a par or as prior to food in a policy of health. They are both good things, but they are not primary.

Muscular energy and activity follow right feeding naturally, and physical training can follow upon the muscular energy. No one indeed disputes this proposition—except in their acts and public policies. There is a general, rather indefinite feeling that sound food is the primary cause of health, but when this shapes itself out of the mist, there appear secondary, not primary, forms—good housing, hygiene, physical drill.

M'Gonigle showed that food took the primary place to good housing and sanitation. Two experiments, now to be recorded, show how food takes the primary place to exercise and physical drill. The first is reported by McCollum and Simmonds.

Forty-two out of eighty-four negro children, in a kindly but impoverished institution, were, as an experiment, given a quart of milk daily in addition to the customary institutional food.

Between these children and the children who were not given milk there was not only a difference of growth and health, but of *desire* for exercise. The non-milk children were apathetic and very tractable. The discipline of the institution was strict, and these children were all obedient. Those in the milk-fed group, on the other hand, soon caused annoyance to their teachers by their restlessness and activity and were frequently guilty of infractions of the rules.

The second human experiment is similar. It can be found in the League of Nations Report on *The Problem of Nutrition*, Volume 1. "A pint of milk daily added to what was considered a good diet in an institutional boarding school" was followed by the usual increased growth and decreased illness, and it was particularly noted "the children were more high-spirited and irrepressible."

The irrepressible activity which good food provides is willingly poured out by the child or man into the many channels that are ready for it. Whether it be as work or play, exercises or drill, sports or sheer necessity, the well-nourished body is glad of the opportunity of activity. Without consciousness of weariness, except if there be lack of variety, this readiness is carried on into age or even near to the time of natural death. Amongst those of excellent physique, getting old has quite a different meaning from what it has amongst those to whom age brings weariness.

So, when the negro and English children showed "restlessness and activity, frequently leading to infractions of the rules," or became "more high-spirited and irrepressible," one sees that more eager activity proceeds from sounder food. One sees, further, that modern urban life, with its industrial and commercial confinement, is, perhaps, only made tolerable by food that is not what the milk was to these black and white boys. The words "apathetic and very tractable" attached to the forty-two negro children who were not given milk are significant. It was food that led to high spirits and infractions of the rules.

Climate is frequently upheld as a cause of disease or of health. McCarrison attributes some of the efficiency of the Hunza to their climate: "No doubt the climate is conducive to the health and vigour which its inhabitants enjoy."

Anyone who has seen the perfect physique of a tiger in the heat of the jungle and, maybe also, of a polar bear in the Arctic, and has watched various races of men in different lands, must, I think, doubt the factor of climate as of great importance in physique and health. Vigorous life is widespread in a world of many climates; there are permanent rainless deserts due to lack of food, but none due to bad climate only.

Finally, in the consideration of the causation of disease, we came to heredity.

We have seen in this chapter that the faith of the medical profession's tenet as to the heredity of tuberculosis has been upset by such human experiments as that of Papworth, so that Varrier-Jones himself stated that the belief was "now generally discredited."

The medical faith goes back at least as far as Hippocrates. It therefore extends over a period of twenty-three centuries. At the modern end of this enduring creed, Karl Pearson brings predestination in the case of tuberculosis into line with the work done generally upon heredity by the words: "the dia-thesis of pulmonary tuberculosis is certainly inherited, and the intensity of the inheritance is sensibly the same as that of any normal physical character yet investigated in man."

Hippocrates was "the Father of Medicine," and Karl Pearson was up to his death, two years or so ago, the greatest British authority on the exactitude of heredity. Can it then be that this faith which has so long been endured and is so buttressed at each end is untrue? And if so, to what degree is heredity as a cause of disease generally untrue?

If a faith has been held so long by a learned profession and yet proves false, it may be that the reason is that it itself lies within the ambit of a yet greater and more widespread human error.

Such an error may well be that of faulty food. It may be that disease is, and for centuries has been, due to faulty food, and because food has been unsuspected, so other faiths have been built up and maintained.

Among these other faiths may be the faith in the inheritance of disease, though it is really only the weakening effect of faulty feeding that is handed on by habit or poverty from generation to generation.

Professor Arthur Thomson, in his well-known book *Heredity* (1926), answers the question he puts to himself : "Can a disease be transmitted?" with this reply : "Perhaps it is best answered in the negative," and he quotes from Professor Martuis : "A disease is not an entity nor a character, but a *process*—an abnormal process injurious to the organism, which is set agoing by a *causa externans* and runs its course in some part of the body. In the sense in which inherited is used in biology *there are no inherited diseases.*"

An *external* cause is necessary.

Certain blemishes and peculiarities are undoubtedly inherited, recurring again and again in one family. Examples of these are : having odd fingers or toes; albinism with whitish hair and pink eyes; pecular movements and mental weakness coming on in middle life, restricted to a very few families and known as Huntingdon's chorea; or the strange inability of the blood to clot, called hæmophilia, which is handed on by unaffected females to their sons.

Nevertheless, there is danger in one's parents. One may be born with a general weakness, and therefore tendency to diseases, due to them.

The hereditary elements are lodged in the sperm cells of the male and the egg cells of the female. Their clusters can be seen under the microscope. There are twenty-four in each human sperm and egg cell. They are called chromosomes and they unite together at the conception of a new human being. But (following the analogy of other living things, for this has not been seen in the human) no sooner does the unity occur than the tiny speck formed by it is separated into two. One of the two bits becomes the reproductive cells of the new being, with their stock of eternal hereditary elements, or genes as they are called, meaning birth-factors or character-factors.

The genes are unaffected by what is going to happen to their tiny companion, which itself will grow into the individual body of the new being.

That being will grow up, unite, and have children, but what he or she does in her lifetime has no effect upon the genes and the intrinsic characteristics which the children inherit through them. That was decided at the first division of the tiny speck.

The genes cannot be changed by the deeds of the individuals who hand them on. They carry with them the imperishable hope of mankind, the indestructibility of the eternal by the temporal. Nevertheless, the temporal *can* cause a general weakness of the genes. It can poison them. It can cause them to be handed on in an enfeebled condition. But it cannot alter their innate characters.

The reason why these genes or birth-factors or character-factors can be weakened is because they dwell in the centres or nucleus of the reproductive cells in the testes or ovaries and are fed by the blood and lymph of the body. Again it is food. They have to be fed. If the food is good, they are strong, if faulty, they are weakened.

Thomson gives some of the causes of the food becoming faulty—excessive alcohol, tobacco, opium, various diseases, "may cause profound changes in the nutritive stream." Still more, of course, can actual faulty feeding of the individual's reproductive cells. So the genes, lodged in the nuclei of these cells, suffer from the unhealthy juices in the cell and are weakened. A general weakness is thus handed on from parent to child, due to the unhealthy ways of the parent. But the parent does not doom the offspring to cancer, tuberculosis, or other particular disease in this way, but only gives it a susceptibility to disease in general. In short, owing to one's parents one can be sickly, but one cannot inherit any specific sickness.

It is this sickliness which results in illnesses which may be caught from the parents or induced by like faulty habits, which are sometimes wrongly regarded as the inheritance of disease or an inherited susceptibility to a particular disease. It is not strictly heredity, for it is due to temporary conditions, and if these temporary conditions are avoided or overcome the illnesses would not occur. Nature endows life with a powerful, eternal capacity to renew itself healthily, given the right conditions. The genes know nothing of diseases.

The primary condition for the health of the future offspring is the proper feeding of the parents so as to provide healthy genes.

I shall not stress further the argument that faulty food is the most general primary cause of disease. But I do wish to stress that it is within the ambit of faulty feeding that at present all the work on human nutrition is being carried out.

In proportion as this is so this work is subjective and carried out in a setting which is not that of health as wholeness. It is studying ourselves and our peoples, amongst whom faulty feeding is innate, and its measures and acceptances of facts are therefore faulty also. It is saturated with a solvent that is itself impure.

To get to the truth it is necessary to be objective, namely, to study health and physique in peoples who have not yet come within the ambit of the faulty feeding of western civilization.

We have to study their food, but much more than their calories, vitamins, proteins, salts, etc. We have to study above all their food's health and its physique, and how these come about, whether its health and physique, both vegetable and animal, completes the circle of health of which it, as the food, is one half and the people who eat it are the other.

Chapter IX

THE HUNZA FOOD AND ITS CULTIVATION

Part I. Food

The foods of the Hunza, as stated in the first chapter, consist of grains, wheat, barley, buckwheat, and small grains; leafy green vegetables, potatoes (introduced half a century ago), other root vegetables, peas and beans; gram or chick pea, and other pulses; fresh milk and buttermilk or lassi; clarified butter and cheese; fruit, chiefly apricots and mulberries, fresh and sun-dried; meat on rare occasions; and sometimes wine made from grapes. Their children are breast-fed up to three years, it being considered unjust to the living child for its lactation to be interrupted by a maternal pregnancy.

The Hunza do not take tea, rice, sugar, or eggs. Chickens in a confined area destroy crops and are not kept.

Looking through the diet, it will be seen that there is nothing strange to the westerner in the Hunza foods. All of them, except perhaps one or two of the smaller grain foods, are common to both peoples.

The difference lies in the *way* they are eaten and the *way* they are cultivated. It is upon these differences that the better health and physique of the Hunza in the major part depends.

Of cereal foods the Hunza prefer wheat, which they themselves grow and which they also get by barter from the Nagiris. Sometimes chick pea is ground up with the wheat, sometimes beans, barley, and peas are ground together. From the wheat-flour they make their bread or chapattis.

This bread is the first of the Hunza foods that differs from the western bread. The Hunza prefers wheat for his bread, so do the English. In this they are alike. But in making it into bread they differ.

The difference is in the grinding. The Hunza grind so that the greater part of the grain appears in the flour. Their resulting bread is wholemeal bread. It is like the Kleiebrot upon which Professor Hindhede fed the Danes, but without the extra bran. It has, of course, its own bran.

The westerners grind their flour to a fine white powder and of this make their bread, which differs from the wholemeal bread in its appearance and its lack of valuable parts of the grain.

McCarrison spoke of the Hunza diet as consisting of "the unsophisticated foods of Nature"; foods not subjected to artificial processes before they reach the consumer. A "sophist" is defined in the English Encyclopædic Dicitionary as "a cunning and skilful man, a teacher of arts and sciences for money." Sophistication for reasons of money does not occur in Hunza.

The Hunza grow their own wheat, but some, as has been said, they get by barter from the Nagiris. They grind it between stones and make their unleavened chapattis from the fresh flour or they take the grain to the mills, where it is made into flour and stored in large chests. They therefore do not eat Nature's foods as they are. Only in the summer do they eat young green corn raw and direct. Otherwise they manipulate it by grinding and cooking.

The westerners do the same. They manipulate and cook their corn to make it into bread. But in their case the term "sophisticated" can be attached to their bread. Art and money both enter into and modify its manufacture.

At one time the British flour was much like the Hunza flour. Then came the introduction of the steam-driven machine, the industrial era and a huge increase of population. More wheat was urgently needed.

In response to this demand the steel-faced plough was invented in America about 1840. This plough solved the problem of grass. Previously grass made a firm matting over the earth, and its removal by hand labour was infinitely tedious. The plough cut up even the tough grass of the prairie and turned the sod upside down so that the exposed roots died.

The virgin soil was exposed, and having the stored soil's food of rotted grass, it yielded excellent crops of wheat. The time came when this store was partly exhausted, but for a long while the wheat-fields answered the hungry call of the increasing manufacturing areas.

The Americans soon erected mills and exported the flour instead of the grain. Now, the part of the grain from which the new plant starts to grow or germ is oily. It is, as one might expect, the part of the grain which best assists the sexual powers of the animal who eats it. It invigorates the whole animal through the strengthening of the reproductive system.

But the wheat germ oil which has this potent effect has a great disadvantage from the point of view of a world trade, such as the opening up of the American prairies offered. If ground up with the flour, the flour was apt to go sour with keeping and on long journeys.

So the germ was eliminated by the commercial milling process.

Covering the wheat grain is a skin—the bran. This protects the grain, as all living skins protect. They all protect in a living way, not merely in a mechanical way like a wall or covering. They can regrow themselves if injured, and beneath and within them they store substances upon which they can call to strengthen their efforts.

In the commercial process of milling this branny skin was also removed. If it stayed behind, it made the flour less white. More of it made the flour brown, and the resulting bread brown bread. Brown bread may be just white flour and bran without the germ, or it may be wholemeal bread, or it may be wholemeal bread with extra bran, like Hindhede's bread.

Whichever it is, it is tinged or coloured. But the new milling turned out a white, or bolted, flour, free of the germ and free of the protective skin, and consisting only of the store, chiefly of starch, set aside in the grain to feed the infant plant. Ground into powder, this made a nice looking white flour which did not go sour with storing, could be carried by trains and ships all over the world and be made into tasty and clean-looking loaves wherever it finally arrived.

But it lacked the supreme vitality area of the grain, the germ, and it lacked the protective skin.

The Hunza bread does not lack these two parts of the grain.

This alone might account for the Hunza's lack of nerves and vigour into old age, for they are great bread eaters. It might also account in part for the sexual disabilities that occur in modern cities and its accompaniments of treatment—commercial nostrums and literature.

Whether this is so or not, the plain fact remains that a part of the grain is thrown away for commercial and æsthetic reasons; that is to say, for sophisticated reasons, from the point of view of food as primary.

There is certainly no instinct in people to guide them to the better bread of the two; for instinct and appetite cannot be regarded as guides in food matters today. They have themselves been so successfully put through the mill of modern commercialism that they have been stripped of reliability. On this point the League of Nations Committee's Report upon *The Problem of Nutrition* declares: "It must be realised that instinct and appetite alone cannot be regarded as reliable guides in the choice of food." And McCollum and Simmonds are more emphatic on this very question of the general acceptance or preference of white flour : *"This (the polishing of rice) and the artificially established liking for white flour and white corn meal,"* they write in italics, *"is an illustration of the failure of the instinct of man to serve as a safe guide in the selection of food.* The æsthetic sense is appealed to in greatest measure in this case by the lowest biologic values."

That original but insufficiently known thinker Mr. Matthias Alexander teaches that the chief defect in modern man is that progress and civilization have proceeded so rapidly that they have outstripped the instincts. The instincts are very slow in their selective formation, and progress has pushed forward at such a speed that it has been impossible for the instincts to keep pace with it. He himself stresses this particularly in the bodily posture, which must impress any observer of urban man. Writing, as I do, in a large public library, the postures of those who are writing amply illustrate Alexander's teaching. They are round-shouldered and ungainly. There is only one writer who I noted wrote with an arrow-straight back, and on enquiry I found that he had been through Alexander's training.

In the matter of food, and particularly in the public favour given to wholemeal bread, this outstripping of the instinct is most noticeable. It is not because wholemeal bread is not tasty. It is a very pleasant bread to the taste, and Hindhede's Kleiebrot is not only tasty but bakes excellently. Nevertheless, men's instincts are not strong enough for its general adoption now, nor were they strong enough to reject white bread at its initial introduction, although, in regard to vitamin B1 alone, the best-fed people of today get less of this vital element than did the parish poor of the eighteenth and early nineteenth centuries.

As Alexander states, if man wishes to regain his pristine health and bodily vigour he has to abandon any reliance on instinct and save himself by knowledge or conscious control.

This can be done by the individual in the matter of bread, for the wholemeal bread is procurable. But to change the habit of the western world is a stupendous task, and one to which its governments have given little attention. For wholemeal bread is a matter of freshness. The Hunza takes his bread fresh from his own fields; we often from great distances, because, though less fresh and vital, it is cheap.

One sees, then, in this respect the value of national self-sufficiency, which has long been a political faith in France and is now one in Germany and has had such an influence on other countries of the west. National self-sufficiency in its principal foods is undoubtedly a necessity, if a nation is to attain to the health that is possible. We who desire to base life on physiology must assert this as an axiom.

It has been said that Britain could not produce enough food for its own people. On the other hand, that great authority Prince Kropotkin calculated that she could produce sufficient food for 100,000,000 people. Anyone who has compared the meticulous care and agrarian economy of China and Japan with the empty grass fields of Britain is forced to the conclusion that the effort to make Britain self-sufficient in food is lacking. In spite of our physiological conviction of the need, the Returns of the Ministry of Agriculture for the last year, ending June 1936, show that progress is still physiological regress. In that year 33,100 more workers were drawn from the land, and this was not caused by mechanisation. No less than 284,900 acres went out of cultivation, 69,000 of these being wheat acres. Potato acreage decreased 7,000 acres. Pigs have decreased by 11,000 breeding sows, cattle by 7,100 head, and chickens to the figure of 884,000. The only increase, possibly in answer to the teachings of the nutritionists, has been in green vegetables, 7,000 acres, and carrots, 1,000 acres.

To sum up, the advantages of the Hunza bread are that it is physiologically economical, for the whole grain is used. Nothing is lost. It is also fresh. It comes from their own fields with the same freshness as fruit and vegetables come from our gardens.

There is one other difference, and that is cultivation. The Hunza, as we shall see in this chapter, have an admirable cultivation. They, moreover, have an irrigation from the mountains, and this spreads a fine silt over the land each year, which is comparable to the silt that is spread over the Egyptian corn-fields by the Nile.

Opposed to this are the prairies of the new world, which yield such magnificent crops in their virginal state. The nitrogen and other nourishment are supplied by the decay of the grass until the steel plough roots up the grass, and destroys it. To them no silt comes annually. After some years of cropping, they have, therefore, to be fed, and they are given chemical manures. There is reason to believe, as will be seen later, that the quality of the grains has deteriorated owing to this. In the recent Lloyd Roberts lecture McCarrison said that in India the same grain, when grown on the same soil and watered in the same way, was of higher nutritive value when the soil had been manured with natural farmyard manure than when manured with artificial chemical manure. It is what one would expect. "Nature," as Dr. Lawrie entitles his iconoclastic book, "hits back."

We all live on milk for a number of months in that period of our lives when growth is most rapid. At that time its freshness is immediate. It has even been shown that this has an unanalysable value, for young animal sucklings do better from breast-feeding than when given their mothers' milk previously withdrawn from the breast.

Milk is therefore a complete food. Adults separate from it the fat as cream or butter, and the proteins as cheese, a protein that is said by nutritionists to have a higher value than that of meat. It is certainly a substitute for meat and largely taken by all agrarian peoples in its place.

Milk has to be fresh. It cannot be transported and stored as flour can. After drawing it stales rapidly, and this constitutes a problem of its supply to those who do not live in the country. In hot countries and seasons, milk is more rapidly affected than in colder ones. Where the cows are liable to tuberculosis, as is the case in western, stalled cows, the milk may convey the disease. Methods to preserve milk are therefore necessary both in the west and east.

In this matter of the preservation of milk it is difficult to say whether the Hunza have the advantage of the west. The Hunza follow the Oriental custom of separating the fat and boiling it to form ghee or clarified butter. They eat the ghee with their food and they use it for cooking. As the boiling forms an intervener between the fresh butter and the consumer, their method cannot be said to be as good as ours. It is in the hot weather forced upon them, for ghee keeps better than butter.

The butter-milk or lassi that is left they drink. They also drink whole milk. They sour milk and butter-milk, which keep better when soured. They take plenty of these liquids with or without spices, though they do not get the large quantities which the Sikhs drink. The souring of milk to preserve it is thus pitted against our method of pasteurization. It is not easy to say which is the better, but the evidence is in favour of the souring, if one accepts the statement that wherever soured milk is largely used—in the Balkans, North Africa and wide areas of Asia—"fine physique, good health and virility are usually seen" (*The Problem of Nutrition*, Vol. I, League of Nations). The contribution to the fine physical development may here be the milk, which these people take much more freely and regularly than we do, and not to any particular virtue in its being soured.

On the other hand, our process of making milk safe has not won general approval.

Firstly, there is the unreliability of milk-pasteurizing plants. Recently in the House of Commons the Minister of Health announced that it was known that a high proportion of pasteurizing plants in London and elsewhere were producing improperly pasteurized milk.

At a later day came a letter to *The Times* from the retiring president of the National Council of Milk Recording Societies, Sir Arnold Wilson, in which he said it had been proved that there was less tuberculosis in rural areas where all milk is drunk raw than in cities where all milk is pasteurized. "Pasteurization," he added "is supported by the whole weight of great commercial interests, who cannot dispense with it, but all available evidence suggests that its value as a safeguard against illness is small."

Moreover, there is evidence that pasteurization reduces certain healthy qualities of milk. Possibly souring does so too. I have found no scientific experiments on this point, and they would have to be very convincing to weigh against the evidence of the Balkan, North African, Arab, Hunza, Sikh, and other drinkers of it with their exceptional physique.

One quality of health which is injured or destroyed by heating, especially if prolonged, is grouped by nutritionists under the vitamin C. So the raising of the milk to 140°F. and keeping it there for half an hour of pasteurization undoubtedly injures it. Wilson quotes the Cattle Diseases Committee as stating that this loss will seriously affect the health of young children if uncorrected by the addition of fruit juice. As lemons and oranges are more expensive that they were, the danger has increased. Anyhow, a method which forces the need of compensating a food is faulty, and part of our "faulty feeding" as the cause of disease. The right way to avoid diseases conveyed by milk is sound human, animal, vegetable and soil nutrition, as Wilson himself concludes.

A further defect of pasteurized milk has been revealed by the work of A. L. Daniels and G. Stearns, published in the American *Journal of Biological Chemistry*, Volume XXXVII (1919). They found by observation that children who were put on milk that was quickly brought to the boiling point and cooled did better in increase of health and weight than children put on the half-an-hour heated pasteurized milk. The reason they gave is that pasteurization leads to the precipitation of the necessary calcium phosphate salts, which can be found clinging to the wall of the container. Whether it was this and the greater loss of the qualities grouped under vitamen C, or some as yet undiscovered cause, does not matter. What does matter is that pasteurization does delimit the health given by milk.

There is another curious fact. Medical officers and the Ministry of Health are both aware that the milk-drinking of the children and people of Britain is too little, and they have provided milk for school children. In most cases this milk is pasteurized. It seems that quite a considerable proportion of children have an aversion to this milk, and get nausea or vomiting, diarrhœa, headache and catarrh, when they take it. The cause, it is said, is not pasteurization, but allergy or exaggerated susceptibility in the majority of cases, and this allergy occurs in children who come from families where there is a similar aversion to milk.

It would be straining the argument to say that this might be instinct in revolt against pasteurized milk in families where instinct for a right food is yet potent, for this point has not been investigated, but I feel sure no such allergy could be found amongst the Hunza and Sikh children. Indian children whom I know never refuse milk.

Both pasteurization and souring are interveners between the fresh milk and the consumer. Of the two the evidence is in favour of souring

We now pass on to leafy-green and root vegetables and pulses. The Hunza, with the exception of their occasional meat, are lacto-vegetarian feeders, such as Hindhede and many other nutritionists, including McCarrison, put as the healthiest diet of mankind. As a general diet it may well be so, though the polar Eskimos, with an entirely opposite diet, do not yield to the lacto-vegetarians in health and physical endurance.

Vegetables therefore play a great part in Hunza feeding. The vegetables they have are mostly similar to ours, but as potatoes, now largely grown and eaten, were only introduced after the British expedition in 1892, they take no part in their traditional well-being.

These vegetables they eat raw when they can, particularly as fuel is scanty. They are fond of raw green corn, young leaves, carrots, turnips, and, as it were to exaggerate their veneration for freshness, they sprout their pulses and eat them and their first green. This eating of sprouting pulse or gram is widespread in Northern India, and undoubtedly within it there is a health which there is not in the pulse itself.

Except for their use of sprouting gram, I do not know that there is any striking difference here. Probably the Hunza eat raw vegetables more freely than we do. Some of us hardly eat them at all, whereas that could not happen among the Hunza.

They have little fuel and small fires. They cook their vegetables chiefly by boiling in covered pots. But the process is more comparable to our way of steaming and cooking in their own juice. Very little water is added. When this has been used up more is added. The water in which the vegetables are cooked is drunk either with the vegetables or later. The point is that it is part of their food. It is not thrown away.

The taking of vegetable water is very obvious sense. It is surprising that we should think that there is nothing soluble in vegetables which is of value, and that they can be soaked and cooked in water without something passing from them into the water. What do pass into the water are salts. Are these salts valuable? The question can be answered by the blunt answer that they are there, and when something is in a food that can be taken, it should be taken. Over and above the fact that a food is a whole thing and should be taken as a whole, there is abundant evidence from the scientists of the loss that occurs through the throwing away of vegetable water of phosphorous, calcium, iron, iodine, sulphur, etc. Quite a considerable proportion of the pharmacopœa seems to have arisen owing to this waste. Quite a considerable number of the doctors' prescriptions and patent medicines may be due to the need to replace the salts of the food in those who suffer from the loss. The similarity of the medicines and the lost salts is too close for one not to be profoundly suspicious that the methods of cooking cause or contribute to the subsequent need of the medicines.

It is not possible to say how this habit of throwing away the water in which vegetables are cooked originated. On the surface it seems clear that it is connected with the plate versus bowl. One cannot drink liquid from a plate. One can only sop it up with bread, and that is wanting in efficiency and manners. But when the food is served in a bowl or bowls, then the fluid part of the food is not lost. I have no doubt that if British children were served their vegetables with the water in which they were cooked in bowls instead of on plates there would be an improvement in their health.

In the culture of their vegetables the Hunza's way differs from that of the west. This vital question will occupy the second part of this chapter. Here it must suffice to say that the Hunza are agrarian craftsmen, individual gardeners, as opposed to rural labourers in large-scale commercial enterprise. So the Hunza vegetables come, as we prefer vegetables to come, straight from the garden.

The Hunza do not wash their vegetables with our assiduity. Like our fondness for white bread, a cleanly appearance appeals to us probably owing to our innate dislike that anyone dirty should handle our food, so we prefer our vegetables very clean. We hate to see them soiled, which may be only due to good, clean earth, but may have other origin. Staining also suggests unhealthiness of the vegetable. Consequently the protective skin of our carrots and other vegetables are apt to be rubbed off, with the result that they decay more rapidly with keeping and their flavours deteriorate. Flavour must be a healthy quality, for it is the bait of nature.

The Hunza eat the edible protective skins of their vege-tables. They do not soak and wash the vegetables to the degree that loses some of the salts as we do, and of course they have no such instruments as those which give celery, for instance, its fine white appearance by getting rid of its valuable outer layers. Their sophistication is far less than ours in this matter too. They, of course, do not eat vegetables dirty as our four-footed brethren are forced to do. They clean to get rid of the soil, but they have no fetish of cleanliness induced by the fear of dangerous dirt as we have.

Meat is a rare pleasure of the Hunza, as it is with the Sikh, both of whom take it on average about every ten days. In Hunza it is scarcer than previously. Some may not get it once a month. It is more frequently eaten in winter. As with the Eskimo and others, the Hunza eat all that is edible of the carcase and not the meat only.

The reason of its scarcity as a food is that the animals are valued as dairy animals in a country where pasture and fodder are scarce. In the winter, when there is still less cattle food, there is more reason for killing.

Animal food is well-liked and figures at feasts. Schomberg describes its cooking on an occasion of ceremony. It is cut up and put into a covered pot with a mass of pounded wheat. Vegetables may also be added and red pepper for seasoning. Very little water is used, and when it is nearly finished more water and vegetables with their juices are added. The vegetables stew in their own juice, the meat and wheat in the water, a slow boiling and steaming like that of the Japanese workers, who make the pot ready in the morning before they go to work, so that the cooking is finished on their return. Schomberg says this slow cooking at ceremonial feasts continues for twenty-four hours. Nothing of course is lost in the material cooked, but such prolonged heat, even in covered pots, must destroy the factors of food, without which scurvy results. The Hunza, however, get no scurvy, because this stew is only a part of their diet and an unusual one. They have ample food to counteract the undoubted faultiness of such prolonged cooking. They also eat sun-dried meat raw, if it is fat and well-flavoured.

This heating, and particularly boiling, is the chiefest human sophistication of food. Its danger is that it destroys the factors grouped round vitamin C, and scurvy, either in its mild form of pallor and lassitude, or its severe form of foul flesh and bleeding, results. Before the cause of scurvy was discovered and better feeding prevented it, it was particularly fatal to soldiers on campaign and men on the high seas. It has been also argued by Mr. A. M. Ludovici in his admirable treatise, *Man's Descent from the Gods,* that the legend of Prometheus can be explained in no other way but by the scorbutic evils which followed the introduction of cooking. Prometheus brought fire to mankind and was punished by Zeus. For in the place of the pristine health of the people came woes and sicknesses, only to be alleviated later by Dionysus, the Saviour, who taught men how to ferment grape juice, ivy juice, honey, and to eat germinated grains. That is the bare outline of this notable explanation, for it is known of course that these fermentations and sproutings, young life in fact, are particularly effective against scurvy. The remedy of Dionysus, in short, was a remedy that would be applied to-day.

Now, at feasts, at Biddulph's "public jollifications," the Hunza drink freely of their fresh home-made wine. So what they lose in the pot they gain from the bottle.

In this the Hunza are followers of Dionysus, as indeed most peasantries have been since the days of the Greek Saviour, if permitted to follow their own bent. The more orthodox teetotal Moslems have, however, long frowned on the Hunza, who, nevertheless, still drink their wine. The Puritans of England, in like manner, frowned upon the English peasants who made merry with the old English ale and mead. Nowadays, the manufactured and advertised products of the brewing and distilling industries have reduced almost to nullity the elderberry, damson, gooseberry, dandelion, applewine and other home-brews of our peasantry.

So, in the matter of balance to cooking by home-brews and sprouting gram, the Hunza undoubtedly are better off than we. Their fermented buttermilk and wines, like their corn from the field and their vegetables from the garden, are direct and lively. They bear freshness with them. They are not staled by interloping.

They therefore fill their original purpose of being valuable for their instrinsic qualities to their creators. Their value may well be that they are a balance of one art against another art, of fermentation against cooking. By fermentation a fresh, living vitality is brought in to balance a food which heat has changed and robbed. That fermented drinks do have to balance something that is lost in cooking has not been proved. It has scarcely been investigated, the question has been so fogged by prejudice. But that fermentation has played a large part in balancing some defect, that, in a cliché, it supplied a long-felt want, seems a very reasonable explanation of the regard which human beings pay to it, even when their food is particularly sound.

"The Hunza are great fruit eaters, especially of apricots and mulberries. They use apricots and mulberries in both the fresh and dry state, drying sufficient of their rich harvest of them for use througout the autumn and winter months" (McCarrison). They eat the fruit fresh in season, cracking the stones and eating the kernels as well. Otherwise they take them, particularly sun-dried apricots, and eat them as they are or rub them in water to form a thick liquid called *chamus*. Dried mulberries they put into cakes as we do sultanas. They do not cook their fruits. "Fruit is really the Hunza staple. It is eaten with bread, far more so than vegetables, as it is more abundant" (Schomberg).

That this fruit is a healthy food is amply proved by the Hunza health. But, then, the Hunza health proves the health of their other foods as well, for it proves a whole. It proves that the foods or diet of the Hunza as a whole result in a human wholeness of health that is supremely excellent. The fruit, forming what Schomberg called the Hunza staple, is clearly therefore good. Everyone, however, is agreed that fresh fruit is excellent. It has a pre-eminence amongst foods which is shown by the words men attach to it—its freshness, its lusciousness, its purity. It is the only food which the average citizen feels comes to him in the intended way, to be accepted in its unchanged natural form. It alone of the foods still preserves its pristine character and therefore is associated in his mind with something of a fresh wholesomeness like the feel of the wind when a new morning breaks. He feels, too, that there is such a direct relationship between the sun and fruit. Fruit, more obviously than other foods, ripens and colours in the sun. Sunlight is the carrier of the sun's quality. Through it that quality comes direct from the great orb of our being. It stores itself in sun-bathed food, as in a minor way electricity is stored in a battery. The eating of fruit releases the sun's quality in its most direct and least interfered-with form.

The Hunza prepare their fruit for the autumn and winter months by drying for a few days in the sun and storing it in baskets in a dry place. Does it thereby gain directly over fruit that is dried and preserved by other processes without exposure to the sun? There is no definite answer to this question. Our storing of fruit is found to lessen its value, but whether there is less loss in sun-dried apricots I have not succeeded in finding in scientific experiment. One can only answer with the old answer—that the Hunza prove their food.

What are the relative amounts of the different foods which the Hunza eat at a meal? This, of course, is left to the individual Hunza. It is a matter of personal appetite and choice.

But, states the report of the League of Nations on *The Problem of Nutrition,* "it must be realised that instinct and appetite alone cannot be regarded as reliable guides in the choice of food."

That is not so with the Hunza. Their instincts and appetites cannot be looked upon as unreliable in relation to their foods. The Hunza still belong to a period when, because sophistication was very limited, instinct was reliable.

Instinct, says Alexander, has been outstripped by the speed of progress. The Hunza have in their mountain isolation kept largely free from that progress. This isolation, however, has been very different from that of the American Indian before the coming European colonists or that of the polar Eskimos, for his country is and has been one of the highwàys between India, Afghanistan, Russia, and China. He has had contact with many peoples. But this has not changed his instinct or culture.

The reason of this is of vital importance in the whole relation of the Hunza to physique and health. The Hunza has not had to follow others. He has, on his part, inherited from immense distances of time a form of agriculture which has claims to be the most successful in the history of man. His agriculture has not been inferior to others. Again, as opposed to American Indians and polar Eskimos, it has been one that is famous far beyond the bounds of his small valley. The valley of the River Hunza, in its way, has possessed and preserved something of the magic of the valley of the River Eurotas.

PART II.   CULTIVATION

The cultivation of the Hunza is that of irrigated, staircase terraces in mountain valleys, and it is probable that it is not only the greatest but it is also the oldest form of agriculture. That is not proven, but it is a growing conviction which Professor Haldane voices in *The Inequality of Man* (1932), that "agriculture started in the mountains, and only later spread to the river valleys."

The importance of the method of culture of food is primary, radical, and fundamental in the matter of health. It exceeds all other aspects of nutrition—if, that is, one separates any aspect of what is a whole. I make no apology, therefore, for asking my readers to leave the Himalaya for a time and transfer themselves to the next mightiest range of mountains, the Andes of Peru. It was in their valleys that the irrigated, staircase farming reached its highest known development.

Twenty years ago the National Geographic Society of the United States sent an expedition to Peru to study the relics of agricultural methods of its ancient people. Mr. O. F. Cook, of the Bureau of Plant Industry of the U.S. Department of Agriculture, was attached as botanist, and he published a report entitled "Staircase Farms of the Ancients" in the Society's magazine of May 1916.

"Agriculture is not a lost art," are his opening words, "but must be reckoned as one of those which reached a remarkable development in the remote past and afterward declined. The system of the ancient Peruvians enabled them to support large populations in places where modern farmers would be helpless."

The system reached its culmination centuries before Columbus discovered America, and before the Incas ruled in Peru. The people who created it have left no written records and bear no historic name. They are, therefore, called after the most striking feature of their work, the megalithic people, because they built the walls of their terraced fields and aqueducts of great stones. These they made to fit, the one with the other, with such accuracy that even to this day they are like those of the Egyptian pyramids, a knife blade cannot be inserted between them.

The megalithic people were great builders with stone. So, following the same traditions, were the Incas. But the work under the Incas was not such a careful fitting, and frequently the interspaces were filled in with clay.

The method of their making of a stairway of terraced fields need not be described. It is much the same as that followed in other mountainous parts, such as, for one, the present Gilgit Agency. The result is a small flat field. Photographed in cross-section, the fields show so many feet of coarse stones and clay below and so many of soil above. The soil was originally imported from beyond the great mountains, for the steep mountain slopes and valleys did not provide it in sufficient quantity. It was refreshed by the silt which the irrigating water brought from the mountains. The soil is still in its place to this day, and to this day each terrace shows the same inside structure whenever walls are removed.

The fields rise up the slopes of the mountains, tier upon

tier, for sometimes over fifty tiers. Some of the walls of the megalithic people are so enormous and well fitted and so formidable in their show of power, that most western travellers have believed them to be fortresses and described them as such, which "only shows how far our own race is from appreciating the devotion of the ancient people to their agricultural pursuits."

Similar fields were built in the valleys themselves. Valley rivers were straightened in their courses and their destructive overflows controlled.

Such were the megalithic achievements in reclamation, besides which, says Cook, in italics, *"our undertakings sink into insignificance on the face of what this vanished race accomplished.* The narrow floors and steep walls of rocky valleys that would appear utterly worthless and hopeless to our engineers were transformed, literally made over, into fertile lands, and were the homes of teeming populations in the prehistoric days." Even to this day thousands of these acres are still fertile and the main support of the native population, who accept them as a matter of course and make no enquiry as to their origin.

The staircase fields were irrigated. The aqueducts were often of great length. Prescott states that "one that traversed the district of Condesuyu measured between four and five hundred miles." Cook publishes a photograph of an aqueduct as a thin dark line traversing a steep mountain wall many hundreds of feet above the valley. It gives one an overwhelming impression of these colossal works, a sudden sense of the stupendousness which is theirs. They were national works, solely for the good of the people. Beside them, as Cook says, the far-famed hanging gardens of Babylon—a pyramid with broad steps of troughs holding soil—was a toy; built, perhaps, to please Nebuchadnezzar's Median queen as a reminder of the terraced culture of her home.

Such works must, one thinks, have supported an agriculture no less wonderful than themselves. This was the case. These Peruvian staircase gardens were a centre, and probably the most important centre, where the agriculture of indigenous American civilizations was created. In them were domesticated and from them were dispersed over the rest of the Americas many vegetable foods.

"The following partial list of the Peruvian crop plants," writes Mr. Cook, "may give an idea of the extent and variety of domestications that were accomplished in Peru: Achupalla (pineapple), anu (Tropacolum), apichu (sweet potato), apincoya (Grandilla), arracacacha (Arracacia), chirimaya, chui (bean), coca (Erythroxylum), cumara (sweet potato), inchis (peanut), oca (oxalis), pallar (Lima bean), papa (potato), papaya, poro (bottle gourd), purutu (frejol), quinoa (Chenopodium), rocoto (Capsicum), rumu (Manihot), sauwinto (guava), sara (maize), tintin (Tacsonia), ullucu (Ullucus), uncucha (Xanthosna), utar (cotton).

"A complete list of the plants that were cultivated by the ancient Peruvians has yet to be made, but it will probably include between seventy and eighty species. A large part are root crops, vegetables and fruits, but some are seed crops, pot herbs, condiments, medicinal plants, dyes, and ornamentals. Annual plants predominate in numbers and importance, but perennials, shrubs and trees are also well represented."

Returning to the Gilgit Agency, one would expect similarities between the conditions of the Andes and north-western Himalaya, both ranges of exceeding loftiness, well-sunned and without excessive rainfall. One would expect these similarities to produce from intelligent peoples a similarity of agriculture.

The agriculture of the valleys of the Gilgit Agency are cultivated by means of terraced fields and irrigation, as were the valleys of ancient Peru.

Further, the area of the Gilgit Agency and its neighbour, the mountainous parts of Afghanistan, once formed an agricultural centre in the same way as Peru. The resemblance of the two greatest mountain areas is very close indeed.

Hunza, which is the best product of the Gilgit Agency, itself is but a microcosm of the Peruvian Empire. In both the people were eager for land, they were in the modern phrase starved for land. Upon their own great efforts depended their continuance as a people in the mountain valleys. So both became distinguished at their best by the arduous perfection of their toil.

It is a most happy fortune that one of the visitors of Hunza was a man who combined artistic sense, historical knowledge, love of mountains, and a sensitive observation in a degree which would be rare in each several faculty. The late Lord Conway explored and climbed both in the Andes and the Western Himalaya.

He was the first to place the redoubtable Hunza in their rightful historic place. "The terraced fields," he wrote, in *The Bolivian Andes* (1901)—Bolivia was a part of Ancient Peru— "reaching aloft, awake vivid reminiscences of the mountain scenery of the north-west frontier of India—as, for instance, in Hunza, where the native population are living in a stage of civilization that must bear no little likeness to that of the Peruvians under Inca government."

In *Climbing and Exploration in the Karakorum Himalaya* (1894), seven years before his visit to the Andes, Conway gave a picture of Hunza which he came to recognize as a microcosm of Ancient Peru. He was on his way to Baltit, the capital of Hunza.

"The path that leads up to Baltit is bordered on either side by a wall of dry cyclopean masonry, the undressed component parts of which are very large and excellently fitted together. Where the slope steepens these walls are placed further apart, and short zigzags are built up between them—a monumental piece of simple engineering. We walked slowly, for there was much to look at, the cultivation being everywhere admirable and each step disclosing some new detail of beauty or interest. The whole of this side of the debris-filled floor of the valley between the cliffs and edge of the river's gorge is covered with terraced fields. They are terraced because they must be flat in order that the irrigating water may lie on them. The downward edge of each terrace must be supported by a strong stone wall, and every one of these is of cyclopean work, like those just described. The cultivated area of the oasis is some five square miles in extent. When it is remembered that the in-

dividual fields average as many as twenty to the acre, it will
be seen what a stupendous mass of work was involved in the
building of these walls and the collection of earth to fill them.
The walls have every appearance of great antiquity, and alone
suffice to prove the long existence in this remote valley of an
organized and industrious community. . . .

"To build these fields was the smaller part of the difficulties
that husbandmen had to face in Hunza. The fields also had
to be irrigated. For this purpose there was but one perennial
supply of water—the torrent from the Ultar glacier. The snout
of that glacier, as has been stated, lies deep in a rock-bound
gorge, whose sides are for a space perpendicular cliffs. The
torrent had to be tapped, and a canal of sufficient volume to
irrigate so large an area had to be carried across the face of
one of these precipices. The Alps contain no *Wasserleitung*
which for volume and boldness of position can be compared
to the Hunza canal. It is a wonderful work for such toolless
people as the Hunzakats to have accomplished, and it must
have been done many centuries ago and maintained ever since,
for it is the life-blood of the valley."

The Peruvians were also comparatively toolless. "That they
should have accomplished these difficult works with such tools
as they possessed is truly wonderful," are Prescott's words.

Conway continues with a brief account of the social system
of the Hunza, which was at his time a miniature of that of the
Incas of Peru. He calls it semi-civilized. I do not think that
is a permissible term. It is a fully developed form of association
of men for their own benefit, supported by tradition and an
accepted form of authority for its execution and adaptation to
any unusual conditions that occur. It is, in a word, a definite
form of agricultural civilization.

"Still more difficult for a semi-civilized people," are
Conway's words, "must have been the elaboration and enforcement of the laws regulating the distribution of the water over
the land. They were a necessity of the situation, and the
existence of the fields proves that such laws were evolved and
maintained. . . . A strong central power, wielded, of course,
by a single hand, was the inevitable result."

We are now able to see with greater clarity and wider observation that the remarkable physique of this people is not causeless nor accidental, nor a happy chance of nature, nor due to fresh mountain air, but that it has a long, long history to support it. It has been famous in its part of the world for its efficiency in the arts of agriculture in the past, it is famous to this day. Its biggest aqueduct, the Berber, is, says Schomberg, "famous everywhere in Asia . . . the mere existence of these kuls (aqueducts) places the men of Hunza as a class apart." They are exceptional agriculturists now, as they must have been in the past, and by that character they have preserved century after century a quality of agriculture which has rendered to them through food its return gift of perfect physique and health. But this they have only maintained through a constant and meticulous devotion to its service.

The agriculture of the north-west frontier of India has been shown to go back into the remotest recesses of human time. What is to be written now cannot be pinned locally to Hunza. Hunza forms a part of the area which it describes. But it is not unfair to think that Hunza, as much as any other part, and possibly more, is a direct descendant from this remote past. All the evidence we have so far produced makes this a reasonable inference.

The evidence is again strikingly like that which Cook produced from Ancient Peru. It is to be found in a report upon *Agricultural Afghanistan,* by Professor N. I. Vavilov and D. D. Bukunich, based on the data and materials of the expedition they undertook for the Institute of Applied Botany. The report was published in Leningrad in 1929. It is in Russian, but there is an English summary of seventy-five pages. An English review of Vavilov's work may also be found in Professor Haldane's essay *Prehistory in the Light of Genetics.* I have followed the English summary published at Leningrad.

Two out of four of the objects of this expedition was (1) to study the different crops and varieties over the slopes of the Hindu-Kush; (2) to study the technique and especially the irrigation of agriculture.

The authors visit "the most typical sedentary farming for

Afghanistan in the narrow high mountain valleys," and note to their surprise: "Nevertheless, this isolated, poor mountain country holds striking riches of varieties, displays an astonishing diversity of the most important crop plants of the Old World."

They give an exhaustive account of the various plants which they found in this area, the many forms of wheat and other cereals, the striking diversity of forms of the beans, peas, and lentils; many forms of salad plants with transitional stages from the weeds to cultivated plants; "multifarious original forms of carrot, turnips and radishes astoundingly rich in varieties"; spinach and other green-leafed vegetables from wildness to cultivation, and finally, "analogical facts revealed by the study of fruit crops: the pomegranate, walnut, apricot, elaeagnus, zizyphus, show features of the primary form originating process."

They thus summarize their conclusions (with their own italics). "The study of the separate crops discussed in the preceding chapters leads us to general geographical conclusions which are in direct connection with the history of agriculture and with the problem of the origin of cultivated plants.

"As the investigation of the varietal diversity of cultivated plants has shown, Afghanistan with the adjacent countries, especially North-western India, is one of the most important primary world agricultural centres, where the diversity of a whole series of plants have originated. This is quite objectively proved *by the varietal diversity of a series of crop plants and by the coincidence of the area of the varietal diversity of many of the most important European crops."*

Thus, as regards the diversity of the important bread-crops, the club and soft wheats, *"Afghanistan occupies the first place among all countries of our planet,"* though "a detailed study of the adjacent north-western India might shift the focus of the origin of forms" (for) "in regard to climate, relief, and crops, the north-western corner of India, immediately bordering on Afghanistan, forms one undivided whole with the latter. The remaining part of the country sharply differs from Afghanistan in climate and soil."

In his studies of the origin of cultivated plants Professor Vavilov found five principal world centres, one of them in south-western Asia. His and his colleagues' detailed investigation of Afghanistan, especially the corner abutting on the Gilgit Agency, has led to a more precise location of the separate crops. "The comparative study of the cultivated plants of Punjab, Kashmir, and the whole of India, have shown that the corner between the Hindu-Kush and the Himalaya must be singled out from the whole of south-western Asia.

"If we turn to the orography and climatalogical maps of India we shall see that its north-western corner is closely connected with Eastern Afghanistan. From the southern territory of India it is separated by the desert Tar; in the north it borders on the Himalaya. Here, in the upper course of the Indus, in Punjab, is concentrated a great diversity of conditions, ranging from the limits of agriculture to sub-tropical conditions; here we find an abundance of water, promoting the development of irrigated cultivation."

The explanation of the exceptional concentration of the primary sources of so many crops of European-Asiatic cultivated vegetation in the largest geological fold of the world is very difficult, say the authors.

The modern Afghans, like the modern Peruvians, simply accept what is left of these ancient gifts, and make no attempt to improve or understand them. On the other hand, unlike Peru, Afghanistan offers no archæological records that throw any light upon this apparently astonishing enigma.

Nevertheless, fortunately, from out of the remote past there loom up some suggestions of a great agricultural race like to the prehistoric Peruvians. "In the last years, in this region (Punjab) connected with Afghanistan, archæological records have been found. These records, synchronical to Mesopotamic culture, remove the beginnings of culture to a much earlier epoch than depicted up to now by history and archæology.

"Henceforward this region, with its diversity of conditions, its concentration of the genes of cultivated plants, its multifarious population, must draw the attention of the investigator. This region evidently holds the keys to many problems of human culture. . . . The concrete solution of this problem will require huge collective work," but, alas, in the contrariness of the modern nations, he sees little hope· of this being made possible in the near present.

In this fold between the Hindu-Kush and the Himalaya lies Hunza. It is, strangely enough, the very bull's-eye of this area. "The Wakhjir pass," writes the *Encyclopædia Britannica* under the heading "Hindu-Kush," "crossing the head of the Taghdumbash Pamir into the sources of the river Hunza, almost marks the trijunction of the three great chains of mountains," the Hindu-Kush, Pamir and Karakoram Himalaya.

Once again one feels the profundity that attaches to the physique of the Hunza people. It is not accident. It is not that of the jungle. It is that of an art, the agricultural art, comparable to the tireless climb by which the Greek architecture finally reached its supreme beauty.

It is in the study of such people that the clue to health is to be found. The final riddle of food and physique lies, not in the laboratories, but in the fields and in such combined research as Professor Vavilov urges.

The final question in the Hunza food thus becomes: Is the circle of health complete? Are the Hunza crops and vegetation as healthy and of as perfect a physique as the Hunza themselves?

The health of their domesticated animals is coupled with theirs. It must also be dependent on the health of the plant growths.

If one takes a modern text-book of plant diseases, such as the well-known *Manual of Plant Diseases* (1935) of Professor Heald of the State College of Washington, one is as appalled by their number as one is by the list of human illnesses in a text-book of medicine. The one is the counterpart of the other.

Heald's list begins with deficiency diseases, nitrogen deficiency, potash and calcium deficiency in tobacco, iron deficiency, magnesium hunger of soya beans, matting of leaves of cereals, grey-speck of oats, yellow berry of wheat, phosphorus deficiency of root crops, potash hunger of potatoes, and so on.

It then passes on to excess diseases. The first of these is nitrogen excess. "Under natural conditions it is rarely present in sufficient quantity to cause injury to our crops, but the amount may be increased to the danger-point by certain farm-cropping practices or by the addition of excessive quantities of nitrogen-containing fertilisers." Then there is the pallor or chlorosis of various plants due to excess of chalk. "Some of these are pear, apple, quince, peach, apricot, prune, plum, cherry, walnut, orange and lemon." There is acidosis and alkalosis—too much acidity, too much alkali. The causes of acidity of the soil are the addition of certain manures, the continued use of acid mineral fertilisers, the interaction of natural residual components of the soil, the removal of lime by plant growth and by leaching through heavy rainfall. Alkali in too great a concentration occurs principally in semi-arid lands. The deeper salts may be brought to the surface by irrigation with the rise of capillary water.

There follow a number of diseases due to some defect in the supply of water, of oxygen to the roots of plants, as in saturated soils, excessive heat or cold, lack of light, the neighbourhood of industrial processes, and diseases due to spraying with chemicals, fumigation, and other forms of over-treatment.

The third great group are the virus diseases. They are infectious diseases due to ultra-microscopic viruses, in the same way as certain human diseases are due to invisible but filtrable viruses.

There follows the great group of parasitic diseases due to microbes, molds, mildews, chytrids, fungi, and finally nematode worms.

How did all these diseases come into being? Were they present or as prevalent in the old agricultural civilizations to which Hunza belongs as they are in our modern civilization? Or are they, too, due to faulty feeding of the plants?

I take it that what has happened to man has happened no less to his domesticated plants. Science has effected a marvellous progress in variety and fragmentation, but at the same time it has torn plants from their traditional conditions upon which their health depends. Plants have been transferred from one locality to another, from one country to another, but the factors of their stable health have not been transferred. Sometimes they have luxuriated in the new wealth of a virgin soil, and then, having wasted its substance, have deteriorated. Sometimes they have met with conditions closely resembling their accustomed ones and have done well. Sometimes all seemed well and then an expected defect showed itself in disease. Sometimes the new conditions brought into being illnesses which were excessively severe. Throughout all their new experiences they have been accompanied by a growing army of plant physicians to enable them to combat the diseases in their severality. There is no doubt, I think, that modern man has made plant life in his own image.

I have been unable to find any history of plant diseases, or study of fossils from this point of view, which could answer such a question, for instance, as: Was the vegetable life of Ancient Peru free from the diseases now current?

In human being one can find some comparison of diseases in the past and now by the examinations, for instance, of the 30,000 bodies of Ancient Egyptians and Nubians which the late Professor Elliott-Smith epitomises in *Egyptian Mummies* (1924). The diseases which would be detected by these belated post-mortems are not numerous, but such as could be detected were found to be very rare, with the one exception of rheumatoid arthritis. Amongst the 30,000 there were three cases of stone in the kidney, one of gallstone, no true case of rickets, syphilis or cancer. There were ten cases of tuberculosis of the bones. Except in the luxury class, there was no caries of the teeth. In the later luxury class caries was as common as it now is in Europe.

But I know of no such study or possible study of plant diseases in the past and now. Nor do I know of any study of plants as they are in a locality where they have long been cultured under like conditions and of the same plants subjected to conditions that are unfamiliar, in which, therefore, their instincts have been outstripped.

Plant life is by its nature less mobile than man's. Movement is only by winged or carried seed, and is limited.

Therefore one would expect the making of plant-life in man's image would have a far more serious effect on plants than on man. Indeed, I sometimes marvel that plants have survived some of the great disturbances to which they have been subjected. It argues much for the scientific skill of man that he should have been able to bring about so many changes at all. But, nevertheless, nature hits back, and she hits back with disease.

From these changes, except for the introduction of the potato in about 1892, the plant-life of Hunza has been exempt.

The unchanged conditions include one of supreme importance, that of food for the plant. This has continued century after century with the utmost constancy.

The chief factors of plant-food have been two.

Firstly, there is the continuous slight renewal of the soil by a sprinkling of the black glacier-ground sand, which is brought to the fields by the aqueducts.

Secondly, there is the direct preparation by man of food for the plants, given in the form of manure.

The Hunza, in their manuring, use everything that they can return to the soil. They carefully collect the cattle manure and store it in the byres. They collect all vegetable parts and pieces that will not serve as food to either man or beast, including such fallen leaves as the cattle will not eat, and mix them with the dung and urine in the byres. They use the human sewage after keeping it for six months. They take silt from special recesses built in their irrigating channels. They collect the ashes of their fires. All these they mix together and make into a compost. They also spread alkaline earth from the hills on their vegetable fields on days when the fields are watered.

The act of manuring is so important in its bearing upon agriculture that the subject needs elaboration. As its classical representatives are the Chinese, it will be their method we will now study. It is to be noted that the Hunza claim to have received culture from Baltistan, the inhabitants of which are Tibetans.

The Chinese have pursued their method of manuring for a period of time which makes modern progress appear an infant, a period which permits the late Professor F. H. King to call his classic of description and understanding by the really stupendous title of *Farmers of Forty Centuries.*

The principle of the method is that of the forest and prairie. It is that everything that comes from the soil, whether it passes through animals or not, is returned to the soil. Nothing is lost, all is preserved. Nothing foreign is intruded, but day by day, year by year, century by century, there is the local transference of death to life again. At one time each piece of matter is dead, but its death is but the awaiting of the time when it will be restored to the living by way of plant food.

The Chinese manure or compost is made of everything that can be collected which once got its life from the soil, directly or indirectly. They are mixed together until they form a black friable substance which is readily spread upon the fields. King describes a number of different processes he saw in different parts of China. One he describes as being carried out in compost pits at the edge of a canal, a process entailing "tremendous labour of body and amount of forethought." Four months before his visit men had brought waste from the stables of Shanghai, a distance of fifteen miles by water. This they had deposited upon the canal bank between layers of thin mud dipped from the canal, corresponding to silt collected in and taken from the recesses in the Hunza aqueducts, and left to ferment. The eight men at King's visit had nearly filled the compost pit with this stable refuse and canal silt. The pit was in a field in which clover, with its peculiar power of taking nitrogen from the air, was in blossom. This was to be cut and piled to a height of five to eight feet upon the compost in the pit, and also saturated layer by layer with canal mud. It would then be allowed to ferment twenty to thirty days, until the juices set free had been absorbed by the winter compost beneath and until the time that the adjacent land had been made ready for the coming crop. The compost would then be distributed by the men over the field.

At another time he saw a compost pit within a village in which had been placed all the manure and waste of the households and streets, all stubble and waste roughage of the fields, all ashes not to be applied directly, mixed up with some soil. Sufficient water was added to keep the contents of the pit saturated and to promote their fermentation. All fibres of organic material have to be broken down, which may require working and re-working, with frequent additions of water and stirring for aeration. Finally the mixture becomes a rich complete fertiliser. It is then allowed to dry and is finely pulverised before it is spread upon the land.

Every foot of land, says King, is made to provide food, fuel, or fabric. "The wastes of the body, of fuel and fabric, are taken back to the field; before doing so they are housed against waste from weather, intelligently compounded and patiently worked at through one, three or even six months, in order to bring them into the most efficient form to serve as manure for the soil or as feed for the crop."

There is no human waste. "While the ultra-civilized Western elaborates destructors for burning garbage at a financial loss and turns sewage into the sea, the Chinese uses both for manure," reported Dr. Arthur Stanley, Health Officer of Shanghai in 1899, and quoted by King. "He wastes nothing while the sacred duty of agriculture is uppermost in his mind. And in reality recent bacterial work has shown that fæcal matter and house refuse" (prepared as it usually is in China in hard-burned glazed terra-cotta urns and in Japan in sheltered cement-lined pits) "are best destroyed by returning them to clean soil, where natural purification takes place. The question of destroying garbage can, I think, under present conditions in Shanghai, be answered in a decided negative. While, to adopt the water-carriage system for sewage and turn it into the river would be an act of sanitary suicide."

The loss caused by the Western systems causes King to utter a powerful anathema against those who wilfully throw away that which is but a part of the cycle of life and death and death and life again. "Man," he cries, "is the most extravagant accelerator of waste the world has ever endured.

His withering blight has fallen upon every living thing within his reach, himself not excepted; and his besom of destruction in the uncontrolled hands of a generation has swept into the sea soil-fertility which only centuries of life could accumulate —fertility which is the substratum of all that is living."

That which is of the soil is best returned to the soil by spreading it as evenly as possible. This was done by the ancient Peruvians, is done by the Hunza, is done by the Chinese and Japanese. All these have great engineering works of irrigation and canalisation. The Chinese spread "the enormous volumes of silt" of their rivers and canals over the land directly as well as a part of their compost. Their huge rivers, as great almost as the Mississipi, sometimes overwhelm them with flood and destruction, but this checks, it never stops, their tireless efforts. Silt and compost must be evenly spread, and so these people take infinite pains to make their land into a series of flat surfaces, "the careful and extensive fitting of fields so largely practised, which both lessens soil erosion and permits a large amount of soluble and suspended matter in the run off to be applied to the fields. . . . If the total area of fields graded practically to a water level in Japan aggregates 11,000 square miles, the total area thus surface-fitted in China must be eight to tenfold this amount. Such enormous field erosion as is tolerated at the present time in our southern and south Atlantic States is permitted nowhere in the Far East, so far as we have observed; not even where the topography is much steeper" (King).

No, nor in Peru nor Hunza, where the topography is of the steepest.

In China, Japan, ancient Peru, Dutch Java, Hunza and other countries, agriculture is a gardening, a care of the soil, a repayment of the soil, carried on by many men and women with never-ending industry.

It is a gardening in which everything that has once had life, even ash and rag, offal and refuse, is brought back to life by the resurrecting power of the soil. The Chinese and Japanese, in following this great principle, prepare and use human excreta, thereby preventing a loss of phosphates alone which King calculates "could not be replaced by 1,295,000 tons of rock phosphate, 75 per cent pure." "The men of Hunza, the most careful and painstaking husbandmen of Asia" (Schomberg), follow the Chinese custom. They have flat fields. They spread out the compost evenly like butter upon bread. They follow, in a word, the garden culture of the immemorial East, and, according to that which Vavilov has found and may yet find, it may perhaps be that it was in their country of the lofty hills that in the distant past this form of compost-culture first came into being in Asia.

It is possible also that in this form of culture there is an excellence of vegetable health which can be obtained by no other means—in Hunza, for example, there is that excellence, and plant disease is insignificant. It is possible that by full repayment to the soil we alone get a full return. It is known that our own agriculture is rather a loan from the soil, for we never repay it in full. We have worked our agriculture on the capital of the soil, and in virgin land we have raided the soil. When the soil sickens we restore it or strive to restore it by scientific doctoring; we return to it in the way of tonics the nitrogen, calcium, phosphorus, of which we have robbed it. Thus disease is patched and mended, but not abolished. The impoverishment of the soil remains our chiefest ill.

For progress, therefore, we now have to look backwards. We have raced forward at too great a speed. We now have to recoil. We have to look back to a period and type of agriculture in which vegetable and animal life were mutually healthy. We have to believe even in the golden age, in which gold did not mean coin in the pocket or blocks in a bank, but an age when the golden sunlight seemed to enter into man through plant and fruit, and bestow the warm gift of health, such an age as the elder Pliny thought upon when he said that for six centuries the men of Rome had needed no physicians.

Chapter X

PROGRESS BY RECOIL

"THE time is not a century distant," wrote King in 1910, "when, throughout the world, a fuller, better development must take place along the lines of these far-reaching and fundamental practices so long and so effectively followed by the Mongolian races in China, Korea and Japan."

We have never had the long tradition of agriculture that we have just described. When England lived only from her land her population was small. It was but five million. There was much land which gave provision for hunting and sport and a plentiful supply of animal food.

We therefore have to recoil, not so much to the ways of our small-peopled country, which was never civilized agriculturally in the full sense, but to countries of longer experience and also of better health.

King frequently inserts into his pages the cheerful, vigorous and healthy appearance of the Chinese lower classes, the Shanghai coolies, "fully the equal of large Americans in frame, but without surplus flesh"; "their great endurance," "both sexes are agile, wiry, and strong" (Hongkong); "lithe, sinewy forms, bright eyes and cheerful faces, particularly among the women, young and old" (Canton); "everywhere we went in China the labouring people appeared healthy and contented, and showed clearly that they were well-nourished." Cheerfulness is, indeed, common to those peasantries who follow the old agricultural ways. Then there is the outstanding example of the Hunza; cheerfulness, however arduous the toil by our measures, however strained the endurance.

The physique and endurance of the Hunza are at present far beyond us as a people, but they are not beyond us by fate. Our genes, our hereditary and eternal capacities, have not been permanently injured and debased. We can recover.

We can recover by knowledge, not by instinct. Our instinct

is no more healthy than we are. But of knowledge we now possess the world in its present and past in a way in which our ancestors never shared or dreamed. So to recover we must recoil; go back to traditions which have been the associates of the food of crowded man for many centuries. This recoil must at present necessarily be fragmental and largely individual. We cannot expect a great agricultural reform movement. Our food fails to figure in our national and political programme in any sufficient, radical and primary way for this to be more than a distant possibility. We have fallen into the way of fragmentation, and by fragmentation, by electicism we must recover. But that fragmentation shall be founded upon the agricultural facts of human people, and not upon those of the laboratory. The laboratory must be ancillary only.

I shall divide the recoil work in this final chapter into its two aspects, general and individual. The general aspect is that of a change or re-adaptation of agricultural methods; the individual aspect deals with what the individual can do for him or herself now to gain better health and physique on the lines indicated by the very healthy people we have studied.

The most important fragment of recoil-work at present occurring in England is one founded upon King's treatise, *Farmers of Forty Centuries,* and first worked out in India at the Institute of Plant Industry, Indore, by the Director, Sir Albert Howard.

Howard and his chief assistant, Mr. Yeshwant D. Wad, in *The Waste Products of Agriculture* (1931), begin their description of their work with the principle that the fertility of the soil is steadily lost by crop production, and must be restored. They review the western, and particularly the dominant New World methods, then pass on to the Far East, quoting freely from Mr. King's book. "In China, fertility has for centuries been maintained at a high level without the importation of artificial manures. . . . In China and Japan, not only the method of soil management, but also the great attention that is paid to systematic preparation, outside the field, of food materials for the crop from all kinds of vegetable and animal wastes, compelled the admiration of one of the most brilliant of the agricultural investigators of the last generation. The results are set out by King in his unfinished work—*Farmers of Forty Centuries*—which should be prescribed as a text-book in every agricultural college in the world."

Howard and Wad collected all the organic material of the farm except the night soil, which, however, has recently been brought into use from the urban neighbourhood; they put them into compost pits, turning and mixing them at regular intervals for aeration as decay proceeded. The Indore process was carried out on a larger scale and with a greater outlay of capital and appliances than the Chinese farmers are able to employ. It was also watched scientifically. But essentially it was the same, a thorough rotting and mixing of organic matter until it was a rich concentrated mixture ready for the new cycle of life.

It is interesting to read amongst the list of the dead waste things that once more become living, in addition to animal manure: cotton stalks, sann hemp (green or dried), pea stalks, sugar-cane stalks, ashes, weeds, and leaves in good quantity; in moderate quantity, dead grass, stumps of millet, sugar-cane and ground-nut, nut husks, wheat straw, and damaged silage; and lastly, these curiosities in small quantities: waste paper, packing material, shavings, sawdust, old gunny bags, old canvas, old uniforms, and old leather belting.

There is in England some land that has the flat surfaces and many water-ways suitable for the older garden-agriculture. Such land is that nearby the Wash; land with a profusion of canals, and such as is richly cultivated by garden-culture in the delta plains of the great Chinese rivers.

At Surfleet, nearby the Wash, in 1935, Captain R. G. M. Wilson changed the method of plant-feeding on his farm of three hundred acres to that of Sir Albert Howard. The results in this Surfleet experiment of but two years' duration have surprised those who have watched it. The vegetables not only have a richer flavour; not only have they a robuster appearance and their leaves a deeper green; not only do they keep better in storage like to that used by the Chinese and Hunza; but in their vegetable health they have attained a new standard. In a paper read by Howard to the Farmers' Club in February 1937 he spoke of the marked improvement in yield and quality of the vegetables, the better tilth and the increased earth-worm population (the Chinese are careful not to injure earth-worms or leave them uncovered by digging). The most striking feature was the general healthiness of the crops and the absence of insect and fungous pests. No chemical sprays have to be called into use. The plants themselves need no such doctoring.

Baron de Rutzen, at the same meeting, related that eighteen months previously he had gone to Holland to observe a similar process. There he had noted "the extraordinary improvement of plant life in quality and in resistance to disease which apparently can be effected by this sort of method," as compared with sprays and other precautionary methods, with which "we had gone to the most absurd lengths."

Mr. Christopher Turnor similarly described his experience in Germany gained from visits paid in the previous two years. The farmers were building up the humus in the soil and abandoning the use of artificial manures.

In Sind, in Rajputana, in the United Provinces, in Assam, the Punjab, in Bihar and Orissa, in Hyderabad, in Travancore, in Ceylon, in Kenya, and in Tanganyika, there are farms and estates in which the Indore methods have proved the same increased health of plants.

All of these experiments are very recent, but it must be remembered that they are not laboratory experiments, but a recoil to principles which have the backing of four thousand years of experience. This is a very different matter from a new discovery. As King says, the Western scientists *discover* things which the farmers of the immemorial East have *known* in practice for forty centuries.

Howard's work in India, in its recoil to primary things, presents a striking parallel to that of McCarrison, or, more accurately speaking, as Howard was the prior worker in the field, McCarrison's work presents the parallel to Howard's. Howard left the conventional way of research and sought for the causes of health in farm vegetables and animals as a whole.

He found diseases to be the indicators of faults due to man himself. McCarrison similarly left the ways of convention and concentrated on the health of the best physical people he could observe. He found diseases to be the indicators of faults due to man himself. In both cases the faults were departures from the primary position of food.

Soon after McCarrison was made Surgeon to the Gilgit Agency Howard was sent out to India as the Imperial Economic Botanist to the Goverment of India. He held the post for twenty years, 1905-1924. He then became Director of the Institute of Plant Industry, Indore, 1924-31.

He had had, of course, a very thorough training in England before being given such an important post. He had already been a research worker in agriculture for six years, but though he had had a laboratory he had never had a farm of his own. In India, at Pusa, he was allotted one of seventy-five acres, "on which I could grow crops in my own way and study their reaction to insect and fungous pests and other things. My real education in agriculture then began."

Pusa was to Howard what Coonoor later became to McCarrison, a place where he had the opportunity and authority of freedom "to try out an idea, namely, to observe what happened when insect and fungous diseases were left alone and allowed to develop unchecked, and where indirect methods only, such as improved cultivation, were employed to prevent attacks."

It is not possible here to describe more fully than has been done these indirect methods. The story of their widening use in vegetable culture, fruit, grains, plantations, and, with the use of clover also in the manner of the Chinese as described by King, in grass pastures for grazing animals, is one of absorbing fascination, which will, it is hoped, soon be put before the public. As an early part of the story which concerns us here it was in Quetta that Howard was given an extra experimental station, 1910-18, and Quetta belongs to the Vavilov area of north-western India, which was described in the last chapter. So it was in Quetta that Howard observed perfect health in fruit trees and their fruits, provided there cultivators carried out the terraced agriculture with thoroughness. As in the case of McCarrison, so also in that of Howard, it was in North-western India that Western observation and Eastern tradition met, and little by little, amongst other principles, emerged the Indore process of compost.

In these years of practical work there was a continuous improvement in the health of Howard's plants and crops. So bold, indeed, did he become in his assurance that by right soil-feeding he had overcome the danger of disease that he offered to import "a supply of the various cotton boll-worms and boll-weevils from America, and the letting of these loose among my cultures. I am pretty certain that they would have found my cotton cultures very indifferent nourishment . . . at Indore during the seven years I was there; I cannot recall a single case of insect or fungous attack."

And what is of the same vital importance as this health of plant life, the animals at Pusa, Quetta and Indore which were fed on the healthy plant-life seemed to take upon themselves the character of the plants. "For twenty-one years (1910-1931)," Howard writes, in "The Role of Insects and Fungi in Agriculture" (*The Empire Cotton Growing Review*, Vol. xiii), "I was able to study the reaction of well-fed animals to epidemic diseases, such as rinderpest, foot-and-mouth disease, septicæmia, and so forth, which frequently devastated the countryside. None of my animals were segregated; none were inoculated; they frequently came in contact with diseased stock. No case of infectious disease occurred. The reward of well-nourished protoplasm was a very high degree of disease resistance, which might even be described as immunity." It will be noted by experts that the resistance covered diseases caused by filter-passing viruses, as well as those due to microbes.

Howard's two principal conclusions in this paper are so important that I have presumed to interpolate some italics. The two conclusions are :

"1   Insects and fungi are not the real cause of plant diseases, and only attack unsuitable varieties or crops improperly grown. *Their true role in agriculture is that of censors for pointing out the crops which are imperfectly nourished. Disease resistance seems to be the natural reward of healthy and well-nourished protoplasm. The first step is to make the soil live by seeing that the supply of humus is maintained.*

"2 The policy of protecting crops from pests by means of sprays, powders and so forth is thoroughly unscientific and radically unsound; even when successful, this procedure merely preserves material hardly worth saving. The annihilation or avoidance of a pest involves the destruction of the real problem; such methods constitute no scientific solution of the trouble, but are mere evasions."

These words, especially those italicized, vividly express, not only the vegetable, but also the animal problem, and not only the animal, but the human.

The secondary conventional causes of disease are not the real causes of disease. Diseases only attack those whose outer circumstances, particularly food, are faulty. The genes of heredity are sound and eternally faithful to healthy life. It is not they who are the givers of disease and of susceptibility to disease, for "disease resistance seems to be the natural reward of well-nourished protoplasm." It is outer causes, not the inwardness of nature, that produce disease. Man is the author of his own destiny.

The prevention and banishment of disease are primarily matters of food; secondarily, of suitable conditions of environment. Antiseptics, medicaments, inoculations, and extirpating operations evade the real problem. Disease is the censor pointing out the humans, animals and plants, who are imperfectly nourished. Its continuance and its increase are proofs that the methods used obscure, they do not attack, the radical problem.

Howard transferred the health of the soil to that of the vegetable, and that of the vegetable to that of the animal, and those of the vegetable and animal back again to the soil.

Transference, transference, transference—three transferences, that is the secret of health. These three transferences —soil to vegetable, vegetable to animal, animal and vegetable back to the soil—form the eternal wheel of health.

We leave this as a fragment of recoil of the utmost importance to our theme of health and physique.

A second recoil is to a part of our own ancestry. Our ancestry of the wealthier classes were great meat eaters and ate few vegetables. The peasants ate grains and vegetables. It was not until Elizabeth's time that melons, gourds, cucumbers, radishes, parsnips, carrots, turnips, and salad herbs, the foods of the "poor commons," came to the tables of delicate gentlemen and the nobility. Much meat food, then as now, was the sign of wealth, and it was the peasantry who followed the principle of "direct to the plant without intermediary," though they, too, fared more richly than the "poor commons" of to-day, having, as small landholders, good bread, brawn pudding, sauce, beef, mutton, shred pies, pig, veal, goose, capon, game, cheese, apples, and nuts.

Their food was raised by means of the open-field system. Of this in England at this day there is but one notable remnant, that of the Isle of Axholme, to which, in 1627, Charles I invited Dutch farmers to drain its marshes and make the land fit for tillage. Their descendants and those influenced by them are the last defence of this ancient system of agriculture. I am not concerned here with the arguments for and against the system of enclosed land which destroyed the open field system, but only with my description.

The Isle of Axholme is flat and hedgeless. Much of the land lies below the level of the tidal rivers, and this low level is used to spread over the land a virgin soil of silt. "In the Isle of Axholme," wrote the late Mr. Rider Haggard, in *Rural England* (1906), "the floods are let on to the land to be treated, which must, of course, lie beneath the high-water level at the rise of the tide, and withdraw themselves through the sluices, leaving behind them a deposit of the thickness and appearance of a sheet of brown paper . . . . A small portion, which lies above the water level has actually been warped (as the process is called) by hand, the mud being let on to it with carts at a great expense from some convenient tidal pool. This, however, was done in the palmy days of agriculture; now no one would dream of incurring such expense."

The result is given by Haggard: "On all the warp lands and some others the crops looked splendid in 1901, especially the wheat and potatoes." Mr. Gilbert Slater, in *The Making of Modern England*, adds this testimony: "Instead of the miserable cultivation for which writers on the subject had prepared me, I saw heavier crops than I had ever seen anywhere else." And in another passage: "Not only are the open fields of the Isle of Axholme exceptionally well cultivated at the present time, but the island also serves as a training-ground in practical and effective farming, and men who begin as labourers there frequently become large farmers elsewhere."

So in the Isle of Axholme there is the spreading of silt, both that suspended in the water and that from the bottom of a water-course, as used by Chinese farmers in their canal districts. The results are excellent. Whether these vegetables also are disease-resistant I have not found out.

A third recoil to be seen in England is the increase of garden-culture seen in the spread of allotments and market-gardening near towns.

Here great opportunities lie. Firstly, these small plots of land could be served by compost-making factories on the model of Howard and Wad's factory at Indore, which supplied such beneficial manure to Indian ryots. This would need a system of co-operation, and co-operation is unfortunately not a habit of English people who work upon the land. It would need co-operation, because the compost itself would have to be compounded from the waste products of allotments, market-gardens and farms, and eventually the towns, and the workers on the land would have to be inspired —there is no other word—by the divine truth that everything that once was living can be returned to the living by the will of man. The result would be to bring a freshness to the vegetable and to the animal food of both the growers and the townsfolk of their neighbourhood, a freshness and flavour which are the witnesses of health.

There is the further problem of the wisdom of the flatness of field surfaces that the compost may be evenly spread. On a question of such engineering magnitude I do not feel it is easy to speak. It clearly needs much understanding and labour on the part of men. It would require much more employment on the land than the land at present provides.

I can only here record briefly how the Hunza solves this problem. The description is one kindly sent to me by Col. Schomberg.

When a Hunza decides to bring a slope of land into cultivation he first digs a ditch horizontally across the slope near the foot of the land to be terraced. He then throws all the stones on the slope, and more, which he transports if need be, to the foot of the slope itself. On this foundation the earth from the trench or hürt is laid. He will then dig another ditch or hürt higher up, also horizontally across the slope, and level the ground in the same manner. When the small fields are level he floods them with irrigation water and silt. The hürt carries off the surplus water, and any leakage which occurs is detected and stopped up, until with further flooding the irrigation-water is held. The cultivator has then succeeded in making a small flat field which holds the water and silt of irrigation.

That brings to an end the general aspect of recoil in England.

We now have to consider the individual aspect. Can the individual in England as it is gain any advantages in health and physique by his practical knowledge of Hunza foods? The answer is undoubtedly that he can do so. A great deal can be done by attention and application of food methods of exceptionally healthy people.

Firstly, it is necessary to convince the individual of its necessity, or at least its desirability. Any man is at liberty, unfortunately, to live a C3 life without any effort to better it. There are so many C3 lives in a C3 nation that this low level is accepted very largely as normal. Let us, therefore, take the picture of a modern man, as drawn by a vivid medical writer, and see if it is at all like what man is intended or could desire to be.

The picture is from the pen of Professor Martin Sihle, Director of the University Medical Clinic of Riga.

He begins with an account of the general undeniable improvements of certain factors or fragments of public health, such as drainage, ventilation, public squares in towns, public baths, heating of public buildings, isolation in the case of infectious diseases, antisepsis, asepsis, and so on.

It would accordingly be natural to expect that "the health of the people (and in particular of those who actually benefit by the hygenic measures) would have reached a height not previously attained. But that is by no means the case. Vainly should we seek evidence that the generation of the last century, i.e. that generation which lived under the protection of the hygienic measures enumerated above, had actually become healthier and more efficient, although hygienic statistics afford conclusive proof of reduced mortality.

"The death-rate has thus diminished, but this fact, as we shall see, has its definite and understandable cause. *But morbidity increases in such proportions as to cause the utmost apprehension. . . .* On the average man attains an unquestionably greater age than formerly, but marked by a more or less pronounced state of ill-health.

"The normal type of a healthy and strong man is embodied in the statues of classical antiquity, in particular among the Greeks, who in great measure succeeded in approximating to the ideal of health. In order to compare himself with the Greek statues, let anyone stand naked before a mirror and attentively observe his mortal frame. He will be horrified to realise how far removed he is from the proportions of the normal type. The glass reveals to him a flat, frequently concave, chest, protruding stomach, especially under the navel, humped drooping back, the upper portion of which is bent, with crooked, misplaced neck and head, falling away shoulders, with prominent shoulder blades, knees with knock-kneed legs, etc. . . .

"Even when we consider the sense organs of our patients, deviation into pathological functioning frequently strikes us. One person is short-sighted, another hears badly, a third has a so-called chronic cold, and cannot breathe properly through the nose, because he is troubled with polypus and swellings. Inadequacies in the functioning of our internal organs play a substantial part. Lungs and heart may be mentioned first. In many people the lung apices function badly; they are anæmic because they are badly ventilated, since, owing to weakness of breathing, the muscles of the chest do not sufficiently rise and fall. Catarrhal symptoms of the bronchial tubes and blocks in the region of the lower lung are also common. At every step one comes upon defective functioning of the heart. The heart is often enlarged and dyspnœa frequently supervenes.

"And the organs of digestion? Few men have them in complete working order. One has too much stomach acidity, another too little. The wall of the stomach is either slack or displays a tendency to painful spasms. One person cannot digest this dish, another that. Pressure in the neighbourhood of the stomach, heart-burn, eructations occur alternately. The functioning of the bowels is for the most part inactive. Besides constipation, swollen stomach, hæmorrhoid troubles are freely complained of. Congestion of the portal vein and swelling of the liver are of daily occurrence; the organs of the stomach are sunken and aggravate the morbid symptoms.

"On the top of these come, finally, the great host of so-called nervous-psychic complaints, hysteria and neurosis. Sleeplessness, migraine, neuralgia, low spirits, all kinds of depression complete the deplorable picture of civilized man."

That is indeed a deplorable picture of the impoverishment of modern civilized man, but one which we know is not untrue.

It is but the final picture of the impoverishment of our soils, an impoverishment forced upon us because we did not possess the almost unimaginable foresight that was needed to feed the rapidly growing urban populations of the industrial era.

Here is a picture of a soil and animal impoverishment from one of the most distant providers of London and other big towns of England. It is taken from Sir John Orr's excellent treatise on *Minerals in Pasture*.

"Munro reports that in the Falkland Islands sheep have been reared and exported for forty years without any return to the soil to replace the minerals removed. During the last twenty years it has become increasingly difficult to rear lambs. The other animals are also deteriorating." The sheep are exported to the United Kingdom, and with them goes the mineral food of the soil which they represent.

This is a typical instance of what is a widespread loss due to the same causes. "The process of depletion," Orr writes, "and the resulting deterioration which shows itself in decreased rate of growth and production, and in extreme cases by the appearance of disease, is proceeding on all pastures from which milk, carcases or other animal products are taken off without a corresponding replacement being made. Accompanying the visible movement of milk and beef, there is a slow invisible flow of fertility. Every cargo of beef or milk products, every ship-load of bones, leaves the exporting country so much the poorer. In many of the grazing grounds of the world this depletion has become a serious economic problem. In Scotland, for example, generation after generation of sheep have been taken off the hills with little compensatory returns. Accompanying the resulting deterioration of the pasture, the stocks tend to be reduced in the rough hill grazings. . . . This process of depletion of the Scotch hills has been going on with increasing rapidity since the time when the produce of the animals, instead of being consumed on the land and therefore returned to the soil, began to be driven off to be consumed in the industrial areas. There are now districts in the Highlands which could not support populations which once lived there, even though the people were willing to accept the standard of living of their ancestors.

"Richardson has recently called attention to the effects of depletion in Victoria. He has estimated that the soil of Victoria has been depleted to the extent of about 360,000 tons of phosphoric acid during the last sixty years, through the removal of phosphates in the exported meat, meal and other animal products, and that nearly 2,000,000 tons of superphosphate would need to be added to the pasture-lands to restore them to the condition they were in about 1860. He attributes malnutrition in stock to the resulting deficiency of phosphorus in the pastures.

"In our own country this process of depletion has been going on for many years, especially in hill pastures, and it is probable that the recognized decrease in the value of hill pastures in certain areas, owing to the increase in the diseases and mortality of sheep, is associated with the gradual process of the impoverishment of the pasture and its soil.

"There is evidence that the same process of depletion has taken place in India. During the years 1920-25 over 520,000 tons of bones have been exported without any compensating return to the soil. The evidence presented before the Royal Commission on Agriculture in India shows that there has been in recent years a marked deterioration in cattle."

McCarrison himself was an emphatic witness to this deterioration, and the need of co-ordination of all forms of research, nutritional, medical, veterinary, and agricultural.

The waste of western civilization is summed up by King in these words : "On the basis of the data of Wolff, Kellner, and Carpenter, or of Hall, the people of the United States and of Europe are pouring into the sea, lakes or rivers, and into underground waters, from 5,794,300 to 12,000,000 pounds of nitrogen, 1,881,900 to 4,151,000 pounds of potassium, and 777,200 to 3,057,600 pounds of phosphorous per million of adult population annually, and this waste we esteem one of the achievements of our civilization."

This waste shows some of the impoverishment of the soil, which is the canvas upon which Sihle painted the poor picture of modern man. The picture is framed in a golden frame. Modern man's achievements in the increase of wealth have been wonderful, but all the while Nature quietly has been revealing the divine laws of life by his physical impoverishment. We hear in these days the cliché of poverty in the midst of plenty, that poverty has become an anachronism. Meanwhile a greater and more radical poverty continually steals upon us and is accepted.

Sufficient has been said, it is hoped, to show that there is a desirability for the individual westerner to pay heed to the food-methods of a people who "still in great measure succeed in approximating to the ideal of health."

The Hunza food comes straight from the garden-field or the hillside. Its freshness is its excellence. In this we can imitate them by using locally-grown or garden vegetables and fruits. If this is impossible we can ask for vegetables from storage in cool cellars. We can ask for them from farms, where their health has been proved as those of Surfleet have been proved in the last two years. We can ask. We shall often get no satisfactory reply. On the other hand, we may get our veget-ables from proper storage and we may learn something about the farm or farms from which we get them. It will be a beginning of knowledge useful to us, but which we have mostly ignored.

Secondly, we can eat young, fresh vegetable food when we have opportunity. Scientists know that it is then that it is richest in minerals. It is then also that it is preferred by the Hunza, and, indeed, by many peoples, as shown with us by our fondness for new potatoes, young lettuces and carrots.

The most valuable form of young green life that the Hunza, in common with so many Orientals, eat is sprouting gram. This is not hard to make, but again there is need of individual trouble for individual gain. Orientals in London usually get their gram (cicer arietinum) from Egypt or India. They soak it for some hours in water, pour off the water, and put it in damp sand in a warm place for twenty-four to forty-eight hours, when the sprouts will appear. They eat it raw without allowing it to dry, with a little powdered ginger or other condiment. The smaller grams are preferred, for the larger gram is hard, so that sometimes the gram and sprout are quickly boiled to soften them, and part of the freshness lost. Wheat and other grains may be used. The sprouting beans of the Chinese emporium in Soho and the several Chinese restaurants in

London are already becoming popular. The sprouts are particularly valuable in winter and early spring, when fresh vegetables and fruits are hard to obtain. It is, for instance, then that they and sprouting onions are sold freely in Oriental bazaars.

As regards bread, the wholemeal bread must be taken. It is not always easy to get, but always can be got with a little trouble. Most people who eat it come to prefer it to white bread. They find more "body" in it.

The Hunza drink milk, especially butter-milk, and in hot weather, when it perishes, they ferment it. Enough has been said about city pasteurized milk to show that one has to take trouble over one's milk-drinking. The same must be said about many of the commercial forms of fermented milk. It is best to ferment it oneself by Metchnikoff's method, with lactic ferment tablets, which can be procured at any chemist. The milk is fermented daily. A little is transferred to fresh or quickly boiled milk for further fermentation, and the rest drunk. In this way one goes on making the milk in a thermos flask or in the warm kitchen, and tablets do not often have to be used. In the country adults drink fresh raw milk.

Like the Hunza, we can drink the water and juices in which our vegetables are cooked. The vegetables can be served to children in bowls with their juice and water. We, inheriting unfortunately a meat-eating tradition, eat off plates, which waste the juices. People do not always want vegetable soup. The cooking in small quantities of water and adding a little more as it gets used, which is the way of the Hunza, makes the quantity of liquid to be taken less.

Vegetables should not be soaked, and so lose their minerals, nor scraped with too much vigour. Some can be taken raw, especially when young. Salads scarcely need any commendation in these days.

As I said above, we inherit a hunter's and pastoral dietary. Our ancestors lived in an island too large for them, which provided plenty of game. The game ate the vegetation, and our ancestors ate the game. "The tables of the thirteenth century were literally loaded with flesh, fish, and fowl; vegetables were so scarce that it was customary to salt them for keeping,"

writes Mr. Synge, in a *History of Social Life in England* (1906),
and he gives a list of the meats at a small mediæval dinner,
which shows that our ancestors were sportsmen, as well as
breeders—boar, swan, rabbit, mallard, pheasant, pig, teal,
woodcock, snipe. With this, as part compensation to excessive
meat, our ancestors were great drinkers of old ale and other
fermented drinks.

From our ancestors, then, we inherit our liking for meat
and for sport, and are not such good vegetarians. We could
not put up with the meat once in ten or more days of the Hunza.
Nor perhaps would the Hunza, could they get more meat,
without foregoing their milk, butter, and curd-cheese. They,
too, were and are great shikaris or hunters of the ibex and
other mountain game, but with the modern firearm there is
now little left to shoot. So the Hunza meat-ration is low, and
he makes up for it by the milk and cheese his animals give
him in place of their flesh. I do not think that the English
will look upon meat once in ten days as desirable. Their
tradition against it is too strong.

As regards fruit and its freshness, we are all of us as one
with the Hunza. Our ancestors neglected vegetables, but not
fruit. They cultivated a great variety of fruits. The peculiarity
of the Hunza use of fruit is the large amount they dry in the
sun and eat pounded up in water as *chamus* almost daily
throughout the year. Dried fruits, dates, figs, and raisins, dried
mulberries and apricots, are all highly nutritious, but I can
find no report on whether sun-drying, to which many are
subjected, adds to their virtue. Dried fruits are easy to get
and should be eaten when fresh fruits are scarce.

The Hunza crack the apricot kernels and eat them. So they
get nutty food.

The Hunza eat any foods to be eaten at one meal. As we
have seen, they stew meat, wheat, and vegetables in one pot.
They, of course, do not have the varied dishes which often
make up our meals. Their meals are far more repetitive. But
they do not follow the rule of another very healthy people,
the islanders of Tristan da Cunha, namely, one meal one food.

Lastly there is the Hunza wine. There is a greater virtue

in fresh home-made wine like the Hunza than in bottled or fortified wine and spirits, but home-brewed wine and old English ale are scarcely procurable.

To sum up, if individually we wish to get some extra health and physique like that of the Hunza, we should remember the following twelve points :

1. See that the vegetables eaten have the repute of healthiness; do not skin them and waste the skins, and do not throw away the juices and water in which they are cooked. (79 per cent of the green vegetables and 99 per cent of the potatoes eaten in Britain are home-grown).
2. Eat garden vegetables and fruit, if procurable, as soon as possible after gathering them, so as to get the peculiar value of freshness.
3. Eat salads and palatable well-stored raw root vegetables.
4. Drink more milk, buttermilk, skimmed milk, and, if palatable, sour milk. (The fresh milk drunk in Britain is exclusively home-produced).
5. Eat less meat, if grain, vegetables, milk, and cheese are taken; eat animal organs and skin as well as the flesh.
6. Eat plenty of fresh fruit when in season.
7. At other times, take dried fruits, preferably sun-dried.
8. Take germinated gram, grain, or beans, especially in winter and early spring.
9. Eat wholemeal bread; to get the *health* of a food, eat the *whole* of it as far as possible.
10. Eat butter and cheese.
11. Drink fresh wine when there is opportunity, or old English ale, if procurable.
12. Do not eat too many different foods or dishes at one meal; simplify.

From these twelve maxims one may choose as the central essentials : wholemeal bread, sprouted gram in the winter and spring, milk products freely, green-leafed and root vegetables, plenty of fruit, and not much meat. That which divides modern people from them is chiefly one thing—ignorance. They do not know that wholemeal bread is so much more healthful than white bread, yet they are anxious for health. They do not know that sprouted gram is one of the most widespread foods in the world in the winter and early spring, the chief period of sickness, yet they are anxious for health. They do not know the great additional health which can be procured by the free use of milk and its products. They still go on with a little milk in their tea. Yet they are anxious for health. They do not know that there is a good protein in wheat, milk, cheese and vegetables, and that meat is not its only source. They hold, by tradition, that meat is the essential food for strength, and they believe eating it in plenty is a part of human wisdom. For they are anxious for health.

Valuable as these deductions from the Hunza are, they are nevertheless fragmentary. The *whole* meaning of this people is something much greater. It is none less than that the perfect physique and health, which we have grown accustomed to regard as the privilege of the wild, and, with rare exceptions, beyond the attainment of civilized man, is not unattainable. It is attainable, if we give the same devoted service to our soil, its health and the health of its production, as for centuries this remarkable people have given to theirs.

Chapter XI

AN ENTIRE EXPERIMENT

THE individual application of the principles of a very healthy people has been given in the last chapter. It is possible, however, to proceed further and apply the principles to a group of people in England, Holland, or some other western country.

The principles may be considered twofold, namely the manufacture and use of humus, and secondly the avoidance of erosion or loss of the soil.

As regards the second principle, the Hunza depend on levelled fields and controlled water supply. Their valley has a little rain and snow, but irrigation constitutes the principal form of the watering of the soil. By its means water gently percolates through the soil and does not wash it away to such a degree that the silt brought is not sufficient to replenish it.

In England, Holland and other countries there are flat fields, and canals in addition to the rainfall. There are also terraced fields in certain mountainous areas of the west. In the United States, "Mangum" and level terraces are constructed by means of special instruments as a measure against erosion. A description of "Farm Terracing," by Mr. C. E. Ramser, will be found in the *Farmers' Bulletin,* No. 1669, of the United States Department of Agriculture.

The prevention of erosion throughout a group-experiment is necessary. No form of soil, however carefully fed, can furnish the substance of the experiment if it is liable to erosion.

The meaning of erosion was succinctly given by Mr. T. C. Chamberlin, geologist of the University of Chicago, at the White House in 1908. The report is from Circular 33 of the U.S.A. Department of Agriculture.

Mr. Chamberlin estimated that the mean rate of the formation of soil from rock was not greater than about a foot in 10,000 years. Yet in a part of Missouri there had been found a rate of erosion which would remove seven inches of tilled soil in twenty-four years. Under grass that amount of erosion would have taken 3,500 or more years.

Mr. C. E. Ramser, in advocating "Farm Terracing" in the United State, wrote of erosion: "It is estimated that erosion removes not less than 126,000,000,000 pounds of plant-food material from the fields and pastures of the United States every year. This is more than twenty-one times the amount removed by crops (5,900,000,000 pounds), according to an estimate of the National Conference Board."

It is, then, essential that the experiment should be carried out upon flat fields protected against erosion.

The Hunza use humus, and, according to the writers of the *Farmers' Bulletin,* No. 22, of the Department of Agriculture of Canada, humus itself is suspect. "Contrary to general opinion," are the writer's words, "humus in a soil appears to facilitate drifting . . . it tends to prevent the soil from forming into clods that are so effective in checking wind action."

Yet the Hunza and the Chinese use humus, but their soils do not suffer from erosion. One way in which they prevent it is the use of silt from their irrigation channels and canals. The other is by keeping an almost continuous cover of plant growth. This cover protects the soil from erosion due to sun, wind, and rain-storm, as the grass protects the soil of the unploughed prairie.

"In China," writes King, "it is very common to see three crops growing upon the same field at one time, but in different stages of maturity—one nearly ready for harvest, one just coming up, and a third at the stage when it is drawing heavily upon the soil." Thus, as in a kitchen garden, the older and higher crops protect the younger. Mulching with straw is also used by the Chinese, as in kitchen gardens.

As regards the cover of crops, which the soil receives through the succession of seasons, King wrote: "Two crops of rice are commonly grown each year in Southern China, and during the winter and early spring, grain, cabbage, rape, peas, beans, leeks, and ginger may occupy the fields as a third or even fourth crop, making the total year's product very large," and he adds else-where: "even the narrow ridges which retain the water are bearing a heavy crop of soya beans."

In this way the very fertility brought by humus protects the soil against erosion by a cover of vegetation comparable to that which humus brings to primeval land.

The Indore compost, made only with the excreta of animals, but otherwise similar to that made by the Hunza, is already in use at Surfleet, in the flat land near the Wash, and on high but level fields at Farleigh Wallop, Hampshire. A similar type of compost is also used in the flat land near Flushing, in Holland. The results, as previously stated, have already been so uniformly good that one can confidently state that the first ingredients of the experiment, namely, the type of agriculture and the healthy soil leading to healthy plant and animal, are now in being in two western countries.

There remains the human ingredient, the final essential factor of the experiment.

What is wanted is a group of families willing to live upon the products of this particular agriculture, eaten, prepared, or stored in the ways already indicated.

In England it would be impossible to impose such a regimen on any group of peoples, so an experiment ordered by authority cannot be considered. The experiment must be voluntary.

There are no doubt families so interested in the problem of health as to be willing to submit themselves to a reasonable experiment, but the experiment is a prolonged one in its wholeness, and though such families could well adopt these foods, they would not form the stable human element required.

The most suitable group would be one composed of families, members of which worked upon land where this agriculture was being practised. They would see the good health of the crops and animals which they themselves helped to rear, and this would give them the necessary faith for submitting to what would have to be an observed experiment. It would be a long one, for it takes its true start at the conception of a being in the womb of a mother fed upon these foods. But its effect upon those not so conceived would quickly be observable, and if notably beneficial, would be of great importance to the present generation and the question of their health.

The experiment must not be too rigid. However desirable,

it would be a mistake to make the experiment too rigid. Certain customary foods, imported into every village, could not be excluded. The demand for them, one expects, would lessen by degrees, owing to the growing appreciation of the quality and value of the home-grown products.

No particular "balancing" of meals, prescribing of diets, attention to vitamins, or other fragmentation would be required. The families would depend upon the completeness and health of the foods they eat, according to their needs and choice.

An experiment with practical results will always arouse interest. If the anticipated success were attained it would stir the talk and observation of neighbouring cultivators.

Though sharing the usual prejudices of mankind, farmers are practical men, eager for good results. Friendly interest might come tardily, but come it would if results were notably good. So also, when mothers found that their children were unusually healthy, they would talk to their neighbours. Through contact the method would spread locally. It would reach the local authorities, and in time they would co-operate by sending parish or municipal refuse to be composted. Thus a practical farming success with its attendant health of soil, plant, animal, and man would spread. The good health of children born into and reared upon the land's products would come later, and the prolongation of the benefit throughout life yet later.

In this re-introduction of old methods many other aspects—financial, political, social, domestic, and so on—would eventually arise. Important as these will be, it is not practical to discuss them now. All that I wish to stress is that the elements of the experiment are at hand and that a beginning has already been made in rural England.

If my essay succeeds it will draw the attention of my readers to this vital work; it will also, I hope, persuade them that a much-needed research is one directed to very healthy people, however remote they may be and however different from ourselves they may seem, if the question of health is to be adequately answered.

A CATALOG OF SELECTED
DOVER BOOKS
IN ALL FIELDS OF INTEREST

A CATALOG OF SELECTED DOVER
BOOKS IN ALL FIELDS OF INTEREST

CONCERNING THE SPIRITUAL IN ART, Wassily Kandinsky. Pioneering work by father of abstract art. Thoughts on color theory, nature of art. Analysis of earlier masters. 12 illustrations. 80pp. of text. 5⅜ x 8½.   0-486-23411-8

CELTIC ART: The Methods of Construction, George Bain. Simple geometric techniques for making Celtic interlacements, spirals, Kells-type initials, animals, humans, etc. Over 500 illustrations. 160pp. 9 x 12. (Available in U.S. only.)   0-486-22923-8

AN ATLAS OF ANATOMY FOR ARTISTS, Fritz Schider. Most thorough reference work on art anatomy in the world. Hundreds of illustrations, including selections from works by Vesalius, Leonardo, Goya, Ingres, Michelangelo, others. 593 illustrations. 192pp. 7⅛ x 10¼.   0-486-20241-0

CELTIC HAND STROKE-BY-STROKE (Irish Half-Uncial from "The Book of Kells"): An Arthur Baker Calligraphy Manual, Arthur Baker. Complete guide to creating each letter of the alphabet in distinctive Celtic manner. Covers hand position, strokes, pens, inks, paper, more. Illustrated. 48pp. 8¼ x 11.   0-486-24336-2

EASY ORIGAMI, John Montroll. Charming collection of 32 projects (hat, cup, pelican, piano, swan, many more) specially designed for the novice origami hobbyist. Clearly illustrated easy-to-follow instructions insure that even beginning papercrafters will achieve successful results. 48pp. 8¼ x 11.   0-486-27298-2

BLOOMINGDALE'S ILLUSTRATED 1886 CATALOG: Fashions, Dry Goods and Housewares, Bloomingdale Brothers. Famed merchants' extremely rare catalog depicting about 1,700 products: clothing, housewares, firearms, dry goods, jewelry, more. Invaluable for dating, identifying vintage items. Also, copyright-free graphics for artists, designers. Co-published with Henry Ford Museum & Greenfield Village. 160pp. 8¼ x 11.   0-486-25780-0

THE ART OF WORLDLY WISDOM, Baltasar Gracian. "Think with the few and speak with the many," "Friends are a second existence," and "Be able to forget" are among this 1637 volume's 300 pithy maxims. A perfect source of mental and spiritual refreshment, it can be opened at random and appreciated either in brief or at length. 128pp. 5⅜ x 8½.   0-486-44034-6

JOHNSON'S DICTIONARY: A Modern Selection, Samuel Johnson (E. L. McAdam and George Milne, eds.). This modern version reduces the original 1755 edition's 2,300 pages of definitions and literary examples to a more manageable length, retaining the verbal pleasure and historical curiosity of the original. 480pp. 5³⁄₁₆ x 8¼.   0-486-44089-3

ADVENTURES OF HUCKLEBERRY FINN, Mark Twain, Illustrated by E. W. Kemble. A work of eternal richness and complexity, a source of ongoing critical debate, and a literary landmark, Twain's 1885 masterpiece about a barefoot boy's journey of self-discovery has enthralled readers around the world. This handsome clothbound reproduction of the first edition features all 174 of the original black-and-white illustrations. 368pp. 5⅜ x 8½.   0-486-44322-1

STICKLEY CRAFTSMAN FURNITURE CATALOGS, Gustav Stickley and L. & J. G. Stickley. Beautiful, functional furniture in two authentic catalogs from 1910. 594 illustrations, including 277 photos, show settles, rockers, armchairs, reclining chairs, bookcases, desks, tables. 183pp. 6½ x 9¼. 0-486-23838-5

AMERICAN LOCOMOTIVES IN HISTORIC PHOTOGRAPHS: 1858 to 1949, Ron Ziel (ed.). A rare collection of 126 meticulously detailed official photographs, called "builder portraits," of American locomotives that majestically chronicle the rise of steam locomotive power in America. Introduction. Detailed captions. xi+ 129pp. 9 x 12. 0-486-27393-8

AMERICA'S LIGHTHOUSES: An Illustrated History, Francis Ross Holland, Jr. Delightfully written, profusely illustrated fact-filled survey of over 200 American lighthouses since 1716. History, anecdotes, technological advances, more. 240pp. 8 x 10¾. 0-486-25576-X

TOWARDS A NEW ARCHITECTURE, Le Corbusier. Pioneering manifesto by founder of "International School." Technical and aesthetic theories, views of industry, economics, relation of form to function, "mass-production split" and much more. Profusely illustrated. 320pp. 6⅛ x 9¼. (Available in U.S. only.) 0-486-25023-7

HOW THE OTHER HALF LIVES, Jacob Riis. Famous journalistic record, exposing poverty and degradation of New York slums around 1900, by major social reformer. 100 striking and influential photographs. 233pp. 10 x 7⅞. 0-486-22012-5

FRUIT KEY AND TWIG KEY TO TREES AND SHRUBS, William M. Harlow. One of the handiest and most widely used identification aids. Fruit key covers 120 deciduous and evergreen species; twig key 160 deciduous species. Easily used. Over 300 photographs. 126pp. 5⅜ x 8½. 0-486-20511-8

COMMON BIRD SONGS, Dr. Donald J. Borror. Songs of 60 most common U.S. birds: robins, sparrows, cardinals, bluejays, finches, more—arranged in order of increasing complexity. Up to 9 variations of songs of each species.
Cassette and manual 0-486-99911-4

ORCHIDS AS HOUSE PLANTS, Rebecca Tyson Northen. Grow cattleyas and many other kinds of orchids—in a window, in a case, or under artificial light. 63 illustrations. 148pp. 5⅜ x 8½. 0-486-23261-1

MONSTER MAZES, Dave Phillips. Masterful mazes at four levels of difficulty. Avoid deadly perils and evil creatures to find magical treasures. Solutions for all 32 exciting illustrated puzzles. 48pp. 8¼ x 11. 0-486-26005-4

MOZART'S DON GIOVANNI (DOVER OPERA LIBRETTO SERIES), Wolfgang Amadeus Mozart. Introduced and translated by Ellen H. Bleiler. Standard Italian libretto, with complete English translation. Convenient and thoroughly portable—an ideal companion for reading along with a recording or the performance itself. Introduction. List of characters. Plot summary. 121pp. 5¼ x 8½. 0-486-24944-1

FRANK LLOYD WRIGHT'S DANA HOUSE, Donald Hoffmann. Pictorial essay of residential masterpiece with over 160 interior and exterior photos, plans, elevations, sketches and studies. 128pp. 9¼ x 10¾. 0-486-29120-0

THE CLARINET AND CLARINET PLAYING, David Pino. Lively, comprehensive work features suggestions about technique, musicianship, and musical interpretation, as well as guidelines for teaching, making your own reeds, and preparing for public performance. Includes an intriguing look at clarinet history. "A godsend," *The Clarinet,* Journal of the International Clarinet Society. Appendixes. 7 illus. 320pp. 5⅜ x 8½.   0-486-40270-3

HOLLYWOOD GLAMOR PORTRAITS, John Kobal (ed.). 145 photos from 1926-49. Harlow, Gable, Bogart, Bacall; 94 stars in all. Full background on photographers, technical aspects. 160pp. 8⅜ x 11¼.   0-486-23352-9

THE RAVEN AND OTHER FAVORITE POEMS, Edgar Allan Poe. Over 40 of the author's most memorable poems: "The Bells," "Ulalume," "Israfel," "To Helen," "The Conqueror Worm," "Eldorado," "Annabel Lee," many more. Alphabetic lists of titles and first lines. 64pp. 5³⁄₁₆ x 8¼.   0-486-26685-0

PERSONAL MEMOIRS OF U. S. GRANT, Ulysses Simpson Grant. Intelligent, deeply moving firsthand account of Civil War campaigns, considered by many the finest military memoirs ever written. Includes letters, historic photographs, maps and more. 528pp. 6⅛ x 9¼.   0-486-28587-1

ANCIENT EGYPTIAN MATERIALS AND INDUSTRIES, A. Lucas and J. Harris. Fascinating, comprehensive, thoroughly documented text describes this ancient civilization's vast resources and the processes that incorporated them in daily life, including the use of animal products, building materials, cosmetics, perfumes and incense, fibers, glazed ware, glass and its manufacture, materials used in the mummification process, and much more. 544pp. 6¹⁄₈ x 9¹⁄₄. (Available in U.S. only.)
                                                            0-486-40446-3

RUSSIAN STORIES/RUSSKIE RASSKAZY: A Dual-Language Book, edited by Gleb Struve. Twelve tales by such masters as Chekhov, Tolstoy, Dostoevsky, Pushkin, others. Excellent word-for-word English translations on facing pages, plus teaching and study aids, Russian/English vocabulary, biographical/critical introductions, more. 416pp. 5⅜ x 8½.   0-486-26244-8

PHILADELPHIA THEN AND NOW: 60 Sites Photographed in the Past and Present, Kenneth Finkel and Susan Oyama. Rare photographs of City Hall, Logan Square, Independence Hall, Betsy Ross House, other landmarks juxtaposed with contemporary views. Captures changing face of historic city. Introduction. Captions. 128pp. 8¼ x 11.   0-486-25790-8

NORTH AMERICAN INDIAN LIFE: Customs and Traditions of 23 Tribes, Elsie Clews Parsons (ed.). 27 fictionalized essays by noted anthropologists examine religion, customs, government, additional facets of life among the Winnebago, Crow, Zuni, Eskimo, other tribes. 480pp. 6⅛ x 9¼.   0-486-27377-6

TECHNICAL MANUAL AND DICTIONARY OF CLASSICAL BALLET, Gail Grant. Defines, explains, comments on steps, movements, poses and concepts. 15-page pictorial section. Basic book for student, viewer. 127pp. 5⅜ x 8½.
                                                            0-486-21843-0

THE MALE AND FEMALE FIGURE IN MOTION: 60 Classic Photographic Sequences, Eadweard Muybridge. 60 true-action photographs of men and women walking, running, climbing, bending, turning, etc., reproduced from rare 19th-century masterpiece. vi + 121pp. 9 x 12.   0-486-24745-7

CATALOG OF DOVER BOOKS

ANIMALS: 1,419 Copyright-Free Illustrations of Mammals, Birds, Fish, Insects, etc., Jim Harter (ed.). Clear wood engravings present, in extremely lifelike poses, over 1,000 species of animals. One of the most extensive pictorial sourcebooks of its kind. Captions. Index. 284pp. 9 x 12.   0-486-23766-4

1001 QUESTIONS ANSWERED ABOUT THE SEASHORE, N. J. Berrill and Jacquelyn Berrill. Queries answered about dolphins, sea snails, sponges, starfish, fishes, shore birds, many others. Covers appearance, breeding, growth, feeding, much more. 305pp. 5¼ x 8¼.   0-486-23366-9

ATTRACTING BIRDS TO YOUR YARD, William J. Weber. Easy-to-follow guide offers advice on how to attract the greatest diversity of birds: birdhouses, feeders, water and waterers, much more. 96pp. 5³⁄₁₆ x 8¼.   0-486-28927-3

MEDICINAL AND OTHER USES OF NORTH AMERICAN PLANTS: A Historical Survey with Special Reference to the Eastern Indian Tribes, Charlotte Erichsen-Brown. Chronological historical citations document 500 years of usage of plants, trees, shrubs native to eastern Canada, northeastern U.S. Also complete identifying information. 343 illustrations. 544pp. 6½ x 9¼.   0-486-25951-X

STORYBOOK MAZES, Dave Phillips. 23 stories and mazes on two-page spreads: Wizard of Oz, Treasure Island, Robin Hood, etc. Solutions. 64pp. 8¼ x 11.
                                                           0-486-23628-5

AMERICAN NEGRO SONGS: 230 Folk Songs and Spirituals, Religious and Secular, John W. Work. This authoritative study traces the African influences of songs sung and played by black Americans at work, in church, and as entertainment. The author discusses the lyric significance of such songs as "Swing Low, Sweet Chariot," "John Henry," and others and offers the words and music for 230 songs. Bibliography. Index of Song Titles. 272pp. 6½ x 9¼.   0-486-40271-1

MOVIE-STAR PORTRAITS OF THE FORTIES, John Kobal (ed.). 163 glamor, studio photos of 106 stars of the 1940s: Rita Hayworth, Ava Gardner, Marlon Brando, Clark Gable, many more. 176pp. 8⅜ x 11¼.   0-486-23546-7

YEKL and THE IMPORTED BRIDEGROOM AND OTHER STORIES OF YIDDISH NEW YORK, Abraham Cahan. Film Hester Street based on *Yekl* (1896). Novel, other stories among first about Jewish immigrants on N.Y.'s East Side. 240pp. 5⅜ x 8½.   0-486-22427-9

SELECTED POEMS, Walt Whitman. Generous sampling from *Leaves of Grass*. Twenty-four poems include "I Hear America Singing," "Song of the Open Road," "I Sing the Body Electric," "When Lilacs Last in the Dooryard Bloom'd," "O Captain! My Captain!"—all reprinted from an authoritative edition. Lists of titles and first lines. 128pp. 5³⁄₁₆ x 8¼.   0-486-26878-0

SONGS OF EXPERIENCE: Facsimile Reproduction with 26 Plates in Full Color, William Blake. 26 full-color plates from a rare 1826 edition. Includes "The Tyger," "London," "Holy Thursday," and other poems. Printed text of poems. 48pp. 5¼ x 7.
                                                           0-486-24636-1

THE BEST TALES OF HOFFMANN, E. T. A. Hoffmann. 10 of Hoffmann's most important stories: "Nutcracker and the King of Mice," "The Golden Flowerpot," etc. 458pp. 5⅜ x 8½.   0-486-21793-0

THE BOOK OF TEA, Kakuzo Okakura. Minor classic of the Orient: entertaining, charming explanation, interpretation of traditional Japanese culture in terms of tea ceremony. 94pp. 5⅜ x 8½.   0-486-20070-1

FRENCH STORIES/CONTES FRANÇAIS: A Dual-Language Book, Wallace Fowlie. Ten stories by French masters, Voltaire to Camus: "Micromegas" by Voltaire; "The Atheist's Mass" by Balzac; "Minuet" by de Maupassant; "The Guest" by Camus, six more. Excellent English translations on facing pages. Also French-English vocabulary list, exercises, more. 352pp. 5⅜ x 8½. 0-486-26443-2

CHICAGO AT THE TURN OF THE CENTURY IN PHOTOGRAPHS: 122 Historic Views from the Collections of the Chicago Historical Society, Larry A. Viskochil. Rare large-format prints offer detailed views of City Hall, State Street, the Loop, Hull House, Union Station, many other landmarks, circa 1904-1913. Introduction. Captions. Maps. 144pp. 9⅜ x 12¼. 0-486-24656-6

OLD BROOKLYN IN EARLY PHOTOGRAPHS, 1865-1929, William Lee Younger. Luna Park, Gravesend race track, construction of Grand Army Plaza, moving of Hotel Brighton, etc. 157 previously unpublished photographs. 165pp. 8⅞ x 11¾. 0-486-23587-4

THE MYTHS OF THE NORTH AMERICAN INDIANS, Lewis Spence. Rich anthology of the myths and legends of the Algonquins, Iroquois, Pawnees and Sioux, prefaced by an extensive historical and ethnological commentary. 36 illustrations. 480pp. 5⅜ x 8½. 0-486-25967-6

AN ENCYCLOPEDIA OF BATTLES: Accounts of Over 1,560 Battles from 1479 B.C. to the Present, David Eggenberger. Essential details of every major battle in recorded history from the first battle of Megiddo in 1479 B.C. to Grenada in 1984. List of Battle Maps. New Appendix covering the years 1967-1984. Index. 99 illustrations. 544pp. 6½ x 9¼. 0-486-24913-1

SAILING ALONE AROUND THE WORLD, Captain Joshua Slocum. First man to sail around the world, alone, in small boat. One of great feats of seamanship told in delightful manner. 67 illustrations. 294pp. 5⅜ x 8½. 0-486-20326-3

ANARCHISM AND OTHER ESSAYS, Emma Goldman. Powerful, penetrating, prophetic essays on direct action, role of minorities, prison reform, puritan hypocrisy, violence, etc. 271pp. 5⅜ x 8½. 0-486-22484-8

MYTHS OF THE HINDUS AND BUDDHISTS, Ananda K. Coomaraswamy and Sister Nivedita. Great stories of the epics; deeds of Krishna, Shiva, taken from puranas, Vedas, folk tales; etc. 32 illustrations. 400pp. 5⅜ x 8½. 0-486-21759-0

MY BONDAGE AND MY FREEDOM, Frederick Douglass. Born a slave, Douglass became outspoken force in antislavery movement. The best of Douglass' autobiographies. Graphic description of slave life. 464pp. 5⅜ x 8½. 0-486-22457-0

FOLLOWING THE EQUATOR: A Journey Around the World, Mark Twain. Fascinating humorous account of 1897 voyage to Hawaii, Australia, India, New Zealand, etc. Ironic, bemused reports on peoples, customs, climate, flora and fauna, politics, much more. 197 illustrations. 720pp. 5⅜ x 8½. 0-486-26113-1

THE PEOPLE CALLED SHAKERS, Edward D. Andrews. Definitive study of Shakers: origins, beliefs, practices, dances, social organization, furniture and crafts, etc. 33 illustrations. 351pp. 5⅜ x 8½. 0-486-21081-2

THE MYTHS OF GREECE AND ROME, H. A. Guerber. A classic of mythology, generously illustrated, long prized for its simple, graphic, accurate retelling of the principal myths of Greece and Rome, and for its commentary on their origins and significance. With 64 illustrations by Michelangelo, Raphael, Titian, Rubens, Canova, Bernini and others. 480pp. 5⅜ x 8½. 0-486-27584-1

PSYCHOLOGY OF MUSIC, Carl E. Seashore. Classic work discusses music as a medium from psychological viewpoint. Clear treatment of physical acoustics, auditory apparatus, sound perception, development of musical skills, nature of musical feeling, host of other topics. 88 figures. 408pp. 5⅜ x 8½. 0-486-21851-1

LIFE IN ANCIENT EGYPT, Adolf Erman. Fullest, most thorough, detailed older account with much not in more recent books, domestic life, religion, magic, medicine, commerce, much more. Many illustrations reproduce tomb paintings, carvings, hieroglyphs, etc. 597pp. 5⅜ x 8½. 0-486-22632-8

SUNDIALS, Their Theory and Construction, Albert Waugh. Far and away the best, most thorough coverage of ideas, mathematics concerned, types, construction, adjusting anywhere. Simple, nontechnical treatment allows even children to build several of these dials. Over 100 illustrations. 230pp. 5⅜ x 8½. 0-486-22947-5

THEORETICAL HYDRODYNAMICS, L. M. Milne-Thomson. Classic exposition of the mathematical theory of fluid motion, applicable to both hydrodynamics and aerodynamics. Over 600 exercises. 768pp. 6⅛ x 9¼. 0-486-68970-0

OLD-TIME VIGNETTES IN FULL COLOR, Carol Belanger Grafton (ed.). Over 390 charming, often sentimental illustrations, selected from archives of Victorian graphics–pretty women posing, children playing, food, flowers, kittens and puppies, smiling cherubs, birds and butterflies, much more. All copyright-free. 48pp. 9¼ x 12¼. 0-486-27269-9

PERSPECTIVE FOR ARTISTS, Rex Vicat Cole. Depth, perspective of sky and sea, shadows, much more, not usually covered. 391 diagrams, 81 reproductions of drawings and paintings. 279pp. 5⅜ x 8½. 0-486-22487-2

DRAWING THE LIVING FIGURE, Joseph Sheppard. Innovative approach to artistic anatomy focuses on specifics of surface anatomy, rather than muscles and bones. Over 170 drawings of live models in front, back and side views, and in widely varying poses. Accompanying diagrams. 177 illustrations. Introduction. Index. 144pp. 8⅜ x11¼. 0-486-26723-7

GOTHIC AND OLD ENGLISH ALPHABETS: 100 Complete Fonts, Dan X. Solo. Add power, elegance to posters, signs, other graphics with 100 stunning copyright-free alphabets: Blackstone, Dolbey, Germania, 97 more–including many lower-case, numerals, punctuation marks. 104pp. 8⅛ x 11. 0-486-24695-7

THE BOOK OF WOOD CARVING, Charles Marshall Sayers. Finest book for beginners discusses fundamentals and offers 34 designs. "Absolutely first rate . . . well thought out and well executed."–E. J. Tangerman. 118pp. 7¾ x 10⅝. 0-486-23654-4

ILLUSTRATED CATALOG OF CIVIL WAR MILITARY GOODS: Union Army Weapons, Insignia, Uniform Accessories, and Other Equipment, Schuyler, Hartley, and Graham. Rare, profusely illustrated 1846 catalog includes Union Army uniform and dress regulations, arms and ammunition, coats, insignia, flags, swords, rifles, etc. 226 illustrations. 160pp. 9 x 12. 0-486-24939-5

WOMEN'S FASHIONS OF THE EARLY 1900s: An Unabridged Republication of "New York Fashions, 1909," National Cloak & Suit Co. Rare catalog of mail-order fashions documents women's and children's clothing styles shortly after the turn of the century. Captions offer full descriptions, prices. Invaluable resource for fashion, costume historians. Approximately 725 illustrations. 128pp. 8⅜ x 11¼. 0-486-27276-1

HOW TO DO BEADWORK, Mary White. Fundamental book on craft from simple projects to five-bead chains and woven works. 106 illustrations. 142pp. 5⅜ x 8. 0-486-20697-1

THE 1912 AND 1915 GUSTAV STICKLEY FURNITURE CATALOGS, Gustav Stickley. With over 200 detailed illustrations and descriptions, these two catalogs are essential reading and reference materials and identification guides for Stickley furniture. Captions cite materials, dimensions and prices. 112pp. 6½ x 9¼. 0-486-26676-1

EARLY AMERICAN LOCOMOTIVES, John H. White, Jr. Finest locomotive engravings from early 19th century: historical (1804–74), main-line (after 1870), special, foreign, etc. 147 plates. 142pp. 11⅜ x 8¼. 0-486-22772-3

LITTLE BOOK OF EARLY AMERICAN CRAFTS AND TRADES, Peter Stockham (ed.). 1807 children's book explains crafts and trades: baker, hatter, cooper, potter, and many others. 23 copperplate illustrations. 140pp. 4⅝ x 6. 0-486-23336-7

VICTORIAN FASHIONS AND COSTUMES FROM HARPER'S BAZAR, 1867–1898, Stella Blum (ed.). Day costumes, evening wear, sports clothes, shoes, hats, other accessories in over 1,000 detailed engravings. 320pp. 9⅜ x 12¼. 0-486-22990-4

THE LONG ISLAND RAIL ROAD IN EARLY PHOTOGRAPHS, Ron Ziel. Over 220 rare photos, informative text document origin (1844) and development of rail service on Long Island. Vintage views of early trains, locomotives, stations, passengers, crews, much more. Captions. 8⅞ x 11¾. 0-486-26301-0

VOYAGE OF THE LIBERDADE, Joshua Slocum. Great 19th-century mariner's thrilling, first-hand account of the wreck of his ship off South America, the 35-foot boat he built from the wreckage, and its remarkable voyage home. 128pp. 5⅜ x 8½. 0-486-40022-0

TEN BOOKS ON ARCHITECTURE, Vitruvius. The most important book ever written on architecture. Early Roman aesthetics, technology, classical orders, site selection, all other aspects. Morgan translation. 331pp. 5⅜ x 8½. 0-486-20645-9

THE HUMAN FIGURE IN MOTION, Eadweard Muybridge. More than 4,500 stopped-action photos, in action series, showing undraped men, women, children jumping, lying down, throwing, sitting, wrestling, carrying, etc. 390pp. 7⅞ x 10⅝. 0-486-20204-6 Clothbd.

TREES OF THE EASTERN AND CENTRAL UNITED STATES AND CANADA, William M. Harlow. Best one-volume guide to 140 trees. Full descriptions, woodlore, range, etc. Over 600 illustrations. Handy size. 288pp. 4½ x 6⅜. 0-486-20395-6

GROWING AND USING HERBS AND SPICES, Milo Miloradovich. Versatile handbook provides all the information needed for cultivation and use of all the herbs and spices available in North America. 4 illustrations. Index. Glossary. 236pp. 5⅜ x 8½. 0-486-25058-X

BIG BOOK OF MAZES AND LABYRINTHS, Walter Shepherd. 50 mazes and labyrinths in all–classical, solid, ripple, and more–in one great volume. Perfect inexpensive puzzler for clever youngsters. Full solutions. 112pp. 8⅛ x 11. 0-486-22951-3

PIANO TUNING, J. Cree Fischer. Clearest, best book for beginner, amateur. Simple repairs, raising dropped notes, tuning by easy method of flattened fifths. No previous skills needed. 4 illustrations. 201pp. 5⅜ x 8½. 0-486-23267-0

HINTS TO SINGERS, Lillian Nordica. Selecting the right teacher, developing confidence, overcoming stage fright, and many other important skills receive thoughtful discussion in this indispensible guide, written by a world-famous diva of four decades' experience. 96pp. 5⅜ x 8½. 0-486-40094-8

THE COMPLETE NONSENSE OF EDWARD LEAR, Edward Lear. All nonsense limericks, zany alphabets, Owl and Pussycat, songs, nonsense botany, etc., illustrated by Lear. Total of 320pp. 5⅜ x 8½. (Available in U.S. only.) 0-486-20167-8

VICTORIAN PARLOUR POETRY: An Annotated Anthology, Michael R. Turner. 117 gems by Longfellow, Tennyson, Browning, many lesser-known poets. "The Village Blacksmith," "Curfew Must Not Ring Tonight," "Only a Baby Small," dozens more, often difficult to find elsewhere. Index of poets, titles, first lines. xxiii + 325pp. 5⅝ x 8¼. 0-486-27044-0

DUBLINERS, James Joyce. Fifteen stories offer vivid, tightly focused observations of the lives of Dublin's poorer classes. At least one, "The Dead," is considered a masterpiece. Reprinted complete and unabridged from standard edition. 160pp. 5$\frac{3}{16}$ x 8¼. 0-486-26870-5

GREAT WEIRD TALES: 14 Stories by Lovecraft, Blackwood, Machen and Others, S. T. Joshi (ed.). 14 spellbinding tales, including "The Sin Eater," by Fiona McLeod, "The Eye Above the Mantel," by Frank Belknap Long, as well as renowned works by R. H. Barlow, Lord Dunsany, Arthur Machen, W. C. Morrow and eight other masters of the genre. 256pp. 5⅜ x 8½. (Available in U.S. only.) 0-486-40436-6

THE BOOK OF THE SACRED MAGIC OF ABRAMELIN THE MAGE, translated by S. MacGregor Mathers. Medieval manuscript of ceremonial magic. Basic document in Aleister Crowley, Golden Dawn groups. 268pp. 5⅜ x 8½. 0-486-23211-5

THE BATTLES THAT CHANGED HISTORY, Fletcher Pratt. Eminent historian profiles 16 crucial conflicts, ancient to modern, that changed the course of civilization. 352pp. 5⅜ x 8½. 0-486-41129-X

NEW RUSSIAN-ENGLISH AND ENGLISH-RUSSIAN DICTIONARY, M. A. O'Brien. This is a remarkably handy Russian dictionary, containing a surprising amount of information, including over 70,000 entries. 366pp. 4½ x 6⅛. 0-486-20208-9

NEW YORK IN THE FORTIES, Andreas Feininger. 162 brilliant photographs by the well-known photographer, formerly with *Life* magazine. Commuters, shoppers, Times Square at night, much else from city at its peak. Captions by John von Hartz. 181pp. 9¼ x 10¾. 0-486-23585-8

INDIAN SIGN LANGUAGE, William Tomkins. Over 525 signs developed by Sioux and other tribes. Written instructions and diagrams. Also 290 pictographs. 111pp. 6⅛ x 9¼. 0-486-22029-X

ANATOMY: A Complete Guide for Artists, Joseph Sheppard. A master of figure drawing shows artists how to render human anatomy convincingly. Over 460 illustrations. 224pp. 8⅜ x 11¼. 0-486-27279-6

MEDIEVAL CALLIGRAPHY: Its History and Technique, Marc Drogin. Spirited history, comprehensive instruction manual covers 13 styles (ca. 4th century through 15th). Excellent photographs; directions for duplicating medieval techniques with modern tools. 224pp. 8⅜ x 11¼. 0-486-26142-5

DRIED FLOWERS: How to Prepare Them, Sarah Whitlock and Martha Rankin. Complete instructions on how to use silica gel, meal and borax, perlite aggregate, sand and borax, glycerine and water to create attractive permanent flower arrangements. 12 illustrations. 32pp. 5⅜ x 8½. 0-486-21802-3

EASY-TO-MAKE BIRD FEEDERS FOR WOODWORKERS, Scott D. Campbell. Detailed, simple-to-use guide for designing, constructing, caring for and using feeders. Text, illustrations for 12 classic and contemporary designs. 96pp. 5⅜ x 8½. 0-486-25847-5

THE COMPLETE BOOK OF BIRDHOUSE CONSTRUCTION FOR WOOD-WORKERS, Scott D. Campbell. Detailed instructions, illustrations, tables. Also data on bird habitat and instinct patterns. Bibliography. 3 tables. 63 illustrations in 15 figures. 48pp. 5¼ x 8½. 0-486-24407-5

SCOTTISH WONDER TALES FROM MYTH AND LEGEND, Donald A. Mackenzie. 16 lively tales tell of giants rumbling down mountainsides, of a magic wand that turns stone pillars into warriors, of gods and goddesses, evil hags, powerful forces and more. 240pp. 5⅜ x 8½. 0-486-29677-6

THE HISTORY OF UNDERCLOTHES, C. Willett Cunnington and Phyllis Cunnington. Fascinating, well-documented survey covering six centuries of English undergarments, enhanced with over 100 illustrations: 12th-century laced-up bodice, footed long drawers (1795), 19th-century bustles, l9th-century corsets for men, Victorian "bust improvers," much more. 272pp. 5⅜ x 8¼. 0-486-27124-2

ARTS AND CRAFTS FURNITURE: The Complete Brooks Catalog of 1912, Brooks Manufacturing Co. Photos and detailed descriptions of more than 150 now very collectible furniture designs from the Arts and Crafts movement depict davenports, settees, buffets, desks, tables, chairs, bedsteads, dressers and more, all built of solid, quarter-sawed oak. Invaluable for students and enthusiasts of antiques, Americana and the decorative arts. 80pp. 6½ x 9¼. 0-486-27471-3

WILBUR AND ORVILLE: A Biography of the Wright Brothers, Fred Howard. Definitive, crisply written study tells the full story of the brothers' lives and work. A vividly written biography, unparalleled in scope and color, that also captures the spirit of an extraordinary era. 560pp. 6⅛ x 9¼. 0-486-40297-5

THE ARTS OF THE SAILOR: Knotting, Splicing and Ropework, Hervey Garrett Smith. Indispensable shipboard reference covers tools, basic knots and useful hitches; handsewing and canvas work, more. Over 100 illustrations. Delightful reading for sea lovers. 256pp. 5⅜ x 8½. 0-486-26440-8

FRANK LLOYD WRIGHT'S FALLINGWATER: The House and Its History, Second, Revised Edition, Donald Hoffmann. A total revision—both in text and illustrations—of the standard document on Fallingwater, the boldest, most personal architectural statement of Wright's mature years, updated with valuable new material from the recently opened Frank Lloyd Wright Archives. "Fascinating"–*The New York Times*. 116 illustrations. 128pp. 9¼ x 10¾. 0-486-27430-6

PHOTOGRAPHIC SKETCHBOOK OF THE CIVIL WAR, Alexander Gardner. 100 photos taken on field during the Civil War. Famous shots of Manassas Harper's Ferry, Lincoln, Richmond, slave pens, etc. 244pp. 10⅝ x 8¼. 0-486-22731-6

FIVE ACRES AND INDEPENDENCE, Maurice G. Kains. Great back-to-the-land classic explains basics of self-sufficient farming. The one book to get. 95 illustrations. 397pp. 5⅜ x 8½. 0-486-20974-1

A MODERN HERBAL, Margaret Grieve. Much the fullest, most exact, most useful compilation of herbal material. Gigantic alphabetical encyclopedia, from aconite to zedoary, gives botanical information, medical properties, folklore, economic uses, much else. Indispensable to serious reader. 161 illustrations. 888pp. 6½ x 9¼. 2-vol. set. (Available in U.S. only.)   Vol. I: 0-486-22798-7   Vol. II: 0-486-22799-5

HIDDEN TREASURE MAZE BOOK, Dave Phillips. Solve 34 challenging mazes accompanied by heroic tales of adventure. Evil dragons, people-eating plants, blood-thirsty giants, many more dangerous adversaries lurk at every twist and turn. 34 mazes, stories, solutions. 48pp. 8¼ x 11.   0-486-24566-7

LETTERS OF W. A. MOZART, Wolfgang A. Mozart. Remarkable letters show bawdy wit, humor, imagination, musical insights, contemporary musical world; includes some letters from Leopold Mozart. 276pp. 5⅜ x 8½.   0-486-22859-2

BASIC PRINCIPLES OF CLASSICAL BALLET, Agrippina Vaganova. Great Russian theoretician, teacher explains methods for teaching classical ballet. 118 illustrations. 175pp. 5⅜ x 8½.   0-486-22036-2

THE JUMPING FROG, Mark Twain. Revenge edition. The original story of The Celebrated Jumping Frog of Calaveras County, a hapless French translation, and Twain's hilarious "retranslation" from the French. 12 illustrations. 66pp. 5⅜ x 8½.
0-486-22686-7

BEST REMEMBERED POEMS, Martin Gardner (ed.). The 126 poems in this superb collection of 19th- and 20th-century British and American verse range from Shelley's "To a Skylark" to the impassioned "Renascence" of Edna St. Vincent Millay and to Edward Lear's whimsical "The Owl and the Pussycat." 224pp. 5⅜ x 8½.
0-486-27165-X

COMPLETE SONNETS, William Shakespeare. Over 150 exquisite poems deal with love, friendship, the tyranny of time, beauty's evanescence, death and other themes in language of remarkable power, precision and beauty. Glossary of archaic terms. 80pp. 5³⁄₁₆ x 8¼.   0-486-26686-9

HISTORIC HOMES OF THE AMERICAN PRESIDENTS, Second, Revised Edition, Irvin Haas. A traveler's guide to American Presidential homes, most open to the public, depicting and describing homes occupied by every American President from George Washington to George Bush. With visiting hours, admission charges, travel routes. 175 photographs. Index. 160pp. 8¼ x 11.   0-486-26751-2

THE WIT AND HUMOR OF OSCAR WILDE, Alvin Redman (ed.). More than 1,000 ripostes, paradoxes, wisecracks: Work is the curse of the drinking classes; I can resist everything except temptation; etc. 258pp. 5⅜ x 8½.   0-486-20602-5

SHAKESPEARE LEXICON AND QUOTATION DICTIONARY, Alexander Schmidt. Full definitions, locations, shades of meaning in every word in plays and poems. More than 50,000 exact quotations. 1,485pp. 6½ x 9¼. 2-vol. set.
Vol. 1: 0-486-22726-X   Vol. 2: 0-486-22727-8

SELECTED POEMS, Emily Dickinson. Over 100 best-known, best-loved poems by one of America's foremost poets, reprinted from authoritative early editions. No comparable edition at this price. Index of first lines. 64pp. 5³⁄₁₆ x 8¼.   0-486-26466-1

THE INSIDIOUS DR. FU-MANCHU, Sax Rohmer. The first of the popular mystery series introduces a pair of English detectives to their archnemesis, the diabolical Dr. Fu-Manchu. Flavorful atmosphere, fast-paced action, and colorful characters enliven this classic of the genre. 208pp. 5³⁄₁₆ x 8¼.   0-486-29898-1

THE MALLEUS MALEFICARUM OF KRAMER AND SPRENGER, translated by Montague Summers. Full text of most important witchhunter's "bible," used by both Catholics and Protestants. 278pp. 6⅝ x 10. 0-486-22802-9

SPANISH STORIES/CUENTOS ESPAÑOLES: A Dual-Language Book, Angel Flores (ed.). Unique format offers 13 great stories in Spanish by Cervantes, Borges, others. Faithful English translations on facing pages. 352pp. 5⅜ x 8½.
0-486-25399-6

GARDEN CITY, LONG ISLAND, IN EARLY PHOTOGRAPHS, 1869–1919, Mildred H. Smith. Handsome treasury of 118 vintage pictures, accompanied by carefully researched captions, document the Garden City Hotel fire (1899), the Vanderbilt Cup Race (1908), the first airmail flight departing from the Nassau Boulevard Aerodrome (1911), and much more. 96pp. 8⅞ x 11¾. 0-486-40669-5

OLD QUEENS, N.Y., IN EARLY PHOTOGRAPHS, Vincent F. Seyfried and William Asadorian. Over 160 rare photographs of Maspeth, Jamaica, Jackson Heights, and other areas. Vintage views of DeWitt Clinton mansion, 1939 World's Fair and more. Captions. 192pp. 8⅞ x 11. 0-486-26358-4

CAPTURED BY THE INDIANS: 15 Firsthand Accounts, 1750-1870, Frederick Drimmer. Astounding true historical accounts of grisly torture, bloody conflicts, relentless pursuits, miraculous escapes and more, by people who lived to tell the tale. 384pp. 5⅜ x 8½. 0-486-24901-8

THE WORLD'S GREAT SPEECHES (Fourth Enlarged Edition), Lewis Copeland, Lawrence W. Lamm, and Stephen J. McKenna. Nearly 300 speeches provide public speakers with a wealth of updated quotes and inspiration–from Pericles' funeral oration and William Jennings Bryan's "Cross of Gold Speech" to Malcolm X's powerful words on the Black Revolution and Earl of Spenser's tribute to his sister, Diana, Princess of Wales. 944pp. 5⅜ x 8⅜. 0-486-40903-1

THE BOOK OF THE SWORD, Sir Richard F. Burton. Great Victorian scholar/adventurer's eloquent, erudite history of the "queen of weapons"–from prehistory to early Roman Empire. Evolution and development of early swords, variations (sabre, broadsword, cutlass, scimitar, etc.), much more. 336pp. 6⅛ x 9¼.
0-486-25434-8

AUTOBIOGRAPHY: The Story of My Experiments with Truth, Mohandas K. Gandhi. Boyhood, legal studies, purification, the growth of the Satyagraha (nonviolent protest) movement. Critical, inspiring work of the man responsible for the freedom of India. 480pp. 5⅜ x 8½. (Available in U.S. only.) 0-486-24593-4

CELTIC MYTHS AND LEGENDS, T. W. Rolleston. Masterful retelling of Irish and Welsh stories and tales. Cuchulain, King Arthur, Deirdre, the Grail, many more. First paperback edition. 58 full-page illustrations. 512pp. 5⅜ x 8½. 0-486-26507-2

THE PRINCIPLES OF PSYCHOLOGY, William James. Famous long course complete, unabridged. Stream of thought, time perception, memory, experimental methods; great work decades ahead of its time. 94 figures. 1,391pp. 5⅜ x 8½. 2-vol. set.
Vol. I: 0-486-20381-6   Vol. II: 0-486-20382-4

THE WORLD AS WILL AND REPRESENTATION, Arthur Schopenhauer. Definitive English translation of Schopenhauer's life work, correcting more than 1,000 errors, omissions in earlier translations. Translated by E. F. J. Payne. Total of 1,269pp. 5⅜ x 8½. 2-vol. set.   Vol. 1: 0-486-21761-2   Vol. 2: 0-486-21762-0

MAGIC AND MYSTERY IN TIBET, Madame Alexandra David-Neel. Experiences among lamas, magicians, sages, sorcerers, Bonpa wizards. A true psychic discovery. 32 illustrations. 321pp. 5⅜ x 8½. (Available in U.S. only.) 0-486-22682-4

THE EGYPTIAN BOOK OF THE DEAD, E. A. Wallis Budge. Complete reproduction of Ani's papyrus, finest ever found. Full hieroglyphic text, interlinear transliteration, word-for-word translation, smooth translation. 533pp. 6½ x 9¼. 0-486-21866-X

HISTORIC COSTUME IN PICTURES, Braun & Schneider. Over 1,450 costumed figures in clearly detailed engravings–from dawn of civilization to end of 19th century. Captions. Many folk costumes. 256pp. 8⅜ x 11¾. 0-486-23150-X

MATHEMATICS FOR THE NONMATHEMATICIAN, Morris Kline. Detailed, college-level treatment of mathematics in cultural and historical context, with numerous exercises. Recommended Reading Lists. Tables. Numerous figures. 641pp. 5⅜ x 8½. 0-486-24823-2

PROBABILISTIC METHODS IN THE THEORY OF STRUCTURES, Isaac Elishakoff. Well-written introduction covers the elements of the theory of probability from two or more random variables, the reliability of such multivariable structures, the theory of random function, Monte Carlo methods of treating problems incapable of exact solution, and more. Examples. 502pp. 5⅜ x 8½. 0-486-40691-1

THE RIME OF THE ANCIENT MARINER, Gustave Doré, S. T. Coleridge. Doré's finest work; 34 plates capture moods, subtleties of poem. Flawless full-size reproductions printed on facing pages with authoritative text of poem. "Beautiful. Simply beautiful."–*Publisher's Weekly.* 77pp. 9¼ x 12. 0-486-22305-1

SCULPTURE: Principles and Practice, Louis Slobodkin. Step-by-step approach to clay, plaster, metals, stone; classical and modern. 253 drawings, photos. 255pp. 8⅛ x 11. 0-486-22960-2

THE INFLUENCE OF SEA POWER UPON HISTORY, 1660–1783, A. T. Mahan. Influential classic of naval history and tactics still used as text in war colleges. First paperback edition. 4 maps. 24 battle plans. 640pp. 5⅜ x 8½. 0-486-25509-3

THE STORY OF THE TITANIC AS TOLD BY ITS SURVIVORS, Jack Winocour (ed.). What it was really like. Panic, despair, shocking inefficiency, and a little heroism. More thrilling than any fictional account. 26 illustrations. 320pp. 5⅜ x 8½. 0-486-20610-6

ONE TWO THREE . . . INFINITY: Facts and Speculations of Science, George Gamow. Great physicist's fascinating, readable overview of contemporary science: number theory, relativity, fourth dimension, entropy, genes, atomic structure, much more. 128 illustrations. Index. 352pp. 5⅜ x 8½. 0-486-25664-2

DALÍ ON MODERN ART: The Cuckolds of Antiquated Modern Art, Salvador Dalí. Influential painter skewers modern art and its practitioners. Outrageous evaluations of Picasso, Cézanne, Turner, more. 15 renderings of paintings discussed. 44 calligraphic decorations by Dalí. 96pp. 5⅜ x 8½. (Available in U.S. only.) 0-486-29220-7

ANTIQUE PLAYING CARDS: A Pictorial History, Henry René D'Allemagne. Over 900 elaborate, decorative images from rare playing cards (14th–20th centuries): Bacchus, death, dancing dogs, hunting scenes, royal coats of arms, players cheating, much more. 96pp. 9¼ x 12¼. 0-486-29265-7

MAKING FURNITURE MASTERPIECES: 30 Projects with Measured Drawings, Franklin H. Gottshall. Step-by-step instructions, illustrations for constructing handsome, useful pieces, among them a Sheraton desk, Chippendale chair, Spanish desk, Queen Anne table and a William and Mary dressing mirror. 224pp. 8⅛ x 11¼. 0-486-29338-6

NORTH AMERICAN INDIAN DESIGNS FOR ARTISTS AND CRAFTSPEOPLE, Eva Wilson. Over 360 authentic copyright-free designs adapted from Navajo blankets, Hopi pottery, Sioux buffalo hides, more. Geometrics, symbolic figures, plant and animal motifs, etc. 128pp. 8⅜ x 11. (Not for sale in the United Kingdom.) 0-486-25341-4

THE FOSSIL BOOK: A Record of Prehistoric Life, Patricia V. Rich et al. Profusely illustrated definitive guide covers everything from single-celled organisms and dinosaurs to birds and mammals and the interplay between climate and man. Over 1,500 illustrations. 760pp. 7½ x 10⅛. 0-486-29371-8

VICTORIAN ARCHITECTURAL DETAILS: Designs for Over 700 Stairs, Mantels, Doors, Windows, Cornices, Porches, and Other Decorative Elements, A. J. Bicknell & Company. Everything from dormer windows and piazzas to balconies and gable ornaments. Also includes elevations and floor plans for handsome, private residences and commercial structures. 80pp. 9⅜ x 12¼. 0-486-44015-X

WESTERN ISLAMIC ARCHITECTURE: A Concise Introduction, John D. Hoag. Profusely illustrated critical appraisal compares and contrasts Islamic mosques and palaces–from Spain and Egypt to other areas in the Middle East. 139 illustrations. 128pp. 6 x 9. 0-486-43760-4

CHINESE ARCHITECTURE: A Pictorial History, Liang Ssu-ch'eng. More than 240 rare photographs and drawings depict temples, pagodas, tombs, bridges, and imperial palaces comprising much of China's architectural heritage. 152 halftones, 94 diagrams. 232pp. 10¾ x 9⅞. 0-486-43999-2

THE RENAISSANCE: Studies in Art and Poetry, Walter Pater. One of the most talked-about books of the 19th century, *The Renaissance* combines scholarship and philosophy in an innovative work of cultural criticism that examines the achievements of Botticelli, Leonardo, Michelangelo, and other artists. "The holy writ of beauty."–Oscar Wilde. 160pp. 5⅜ x 8½. 0-486-44025-7

A TREATISE ON PAINTING, Leonardo da Vinci. The great Renaissance artist's practical advice on drawing and painting techniques covers anatomy, perspective, composition, light and shadow, and color. A classic of art instruction, it features 48 drawings by Nicholas Poussin and Leon Battista Alberti. 192pp. 5⅜ x 8½. 0-486-44155-5

THE MIND OF LEONARDO DA VINCI, Edward McCurdy. More than just a biography, this classic study by a distinguished historian draws upon Leonardo's extensive writings to offer numerous demonstrations of the Renaissance master's achievements, not only in sculpture and painting, but also in music, engineering, and even experimental aviation. 384pp. 5⅜ x 8½. 0-486-44142-3

WASHINGTON IRVING'S RIP VAN WINKLE, Illustrated by Arthur Rackham. Lovely prints that established artist as a leading illustrator of the time and forever etched into the popular imagination a classic of Catskill lore. 51 full-color plates. 80pp. 8⅜ x 11. 0-486-44242-X

HENSCHE ON PAINTING, John W. Robichaux. Basic painting philosophy and methodology of a great teacher, as expounded in his famous classes and workshops on Cape Cod. 7 illustrations in color on covers. 80pp. 5⅜ x 8½. 0-486-43728-0

CATALOG OF DOVER BOOKS

LIGHT AND SHADE: A Classic Approach to Three-Dimensional Drawing, Mrs. Mary P. Merrifield. Handy reference clearly demonstrates principles of light and shade by revealing effects of common daylight, sunshine, and candle or artificial light on geometrical solids. 13 plates. 64pp. 5⅜ x 8½. 0-486-44143-1

ASTROLOGY AND ASTRONOMY: A Pictorial Archive of Signs and Symbols, Ernst and Johanna Lehner. Treasure trove of stories, lore, and myth, accompanied by more than 300 rare illustrations of planets, the Milky Way, signs of the zodiac, comets, meteors, and other astronomical phenomena. 192pp. 8¾ x 11. 0-486-43981-X

JEWELRY MAKING: Techniques for Metal, Tim McCreight. Easy-to-follow instructions and carefully executed illustrations describe tools and techniques, use of gems and enamels, wire inlay, casting, and other topics. 72 line illustrations and diagrams. 176pp. 8¼ x 10⅞. 0-486-44043-5

MAKING BIRDHOUSES: Easy and Advanced Projects, Gladstone Califf. Easy-to-follow instructions include diagrams for everything from a one-room house for bluebirds to a forty-two-room structure for purple martins. 56 plates; 4 figures. 80pp. 8¾ x 6⅝. 0-486-44183-0

LITTLE BOOK OF LOG CABINS: How to Build and Furnish Them, William S. Wicks. Handy how-to manual, with instructions and illustrations for building cabins in the Adirondack style, fireplaces, stairways, furniture, beamed ceilings, and more. 102 line drawings. 96pp. 8¾ x 6⅝. 0-486-44259-4

THE SEASONS OF AMERICA PAST, Eric Sloane. From "sugaring time" and strawberry picking to Indian summer and fall harvest, a whole year's activities described in charming prose and enhanced with 79 of the author's own illustrations. 160pp. 8¼ x 11. 0-486-44220-9

THE METROPOLIS OF TOMORROW, Hugh Ferriss. Generous, prophetic vision of the metropolis of the future, as perceived in 1929. Powerful illustrations of towering structures, wide avenues, and rooftop parks—all features in many of today's modern cities. 59 illustrations. 144pp. 8¼ x 11. 0-486-43727-2

THE PATH TO ROME, Hilaire Belloc. This 1902 memoir abounds in lively vignettes from a vanished time, recounting a pilgrimage on foot across the Alps and Apennines in order to "see all Europe which the Christian Faith has saved." 77 of the author's original line drawings complement his sparkling prose. 272pp. 5⅜ x 8½. 0-486-44001-X

THE HISTORY OF RASSELAS: Prince of Abissinia, Samuel Johnson. Distinguished English writer attacks eighteenth-century optimism and man's unrealistic estimates of what life has to offer. 112pp. 5⅜ x 8½. 0-486-44094-X

A VOYAGE TO ARCTURUS, David Lindsay. A brilliant flight of pure fancy, where wild creatures crowd the fantastic landscape and demented torturers dominate victims with their bizarre mental powers. 272pp. 5⅜ x 8½. 0-486-44198-9

Paperbound unless otherwise indicated. Available at your book dealer, online at **www.doverpublications.com**, or by writing to Dept. GI, Dover Publications, Inc., 31 East 2nd Street, Mineola, NY 11501. For current price information or for free catalogs (please indicate field of interest), write to Dover Publications or log on to **www.doverpublications.com** and see every Dover book in print. Dover publishes more than 500 books each year on science, elementary and advanced mathematics, biology, music, art, literary history, social sciences, and other areas.